Dynamic Materia Medica
Syphilis

A Study of the Syphilitic Miasm through Remedies

Dynamic Materia Medica
Syphilis

A Study of the Syphilitic Miasm through Remedies

Jeremy Yaakov Sherr

Dedicated to James Tyler Kent, genius of homœopathy

It takes courage
to do what you want.

Other people
have a lot of plans for you.

Nobody wants you to do
what you want to do.

They want you to go on their trip,
but you can do what you want.

Joseph Campbell

Dynamic Materia Medica – Syphilis

A Study of the Syphilitic Miasm through Remedies

ISBN number 1 901147 04 5

Published by Dynamis Books
Design – Court Street Design

Printed by
Biddles Limited
Woodbridge Park Estate
Woodbridge Road
Guildford
Surrey GU1 1DA
England

Credits:

"Thallium," "Thallium Toxicology," "Repertory of Thallium Salts Toxicology" and "Syphilis The Disease" written by Tina Quirk; initiated and edited by Jeremy Sherr.

Acknowledgements

Two dear friends, Lani Foulger and Tina Quirk have put an enormous amount of love and work into this volume. They have both dedicated their time, talent and goodwill into making this book possible.

Tina has spent many months editing and proofreading this book and has been a wonderful support throughout its writing. She has scanned the literature and collected substantial amounts of useful information. She has researched and written the chapter 'Syphilis – The Disease' and has collated and researched the toxicology of Thallium. Her love of work and quality complement her love of homoeopathy.

Lani has provided me with the best challenge that a proofreader and editor can offer. She did not let me get away with anything that I should not get away with. Yet she offered her excellent advice in the most patient and homoeopathic manner, teaching me to perceive and correct my own mistakes. And once in a while, a gold star kept me going. Her excellent supervision has done much to improve the quality of this work.

I offer them both my deepest gratitude.

Special thanks to Jake Kiakahi for the missing gene and excellent advice.

Many friends, students and teachers have contributed, knowingly and unknowingly, directly and indirectly, to bringing this book to light. I thank them all.

My students have been my teachers, allowing me to reflect their knowledge as if one person. Thank you Dynamis people.

I thank all my homœopathic teachers for all their precious gifts of knowledge. In particular I would like to thank three teachers who have empowered me with quantum leaps in my homœopathic understanding. Joseph Reves from Israel for philosophy and 'the circle of elements', Vega Rozenberg from Israel for his brilliance and Arnt Faulkman from Norway for planting the seeds of 'the verb'. I also wish to thank Jan Scholten for his periodic table insights.

I would like to thank the following people for their contributions:

The provers of Androctonus and Haliaeetus.
Roger and Clair Ash Wheeler for their faith and support.
Neil Blowers for professionalism and creativity with the layout.
Vera Externest for Phytolacca.
Silvie for universal channels.
Stanley Fefferman for education and encouragement.
Erica Abney and Sarah Heal for research on thallium.
Gill Scot for Guaiacum and Fracastoro.
Mary Gooch and Gabriella Reiberer for Platina research.
Ed and Nancy Zorensky, Marybeth Moseman, Dominique Sorrente, Sandi Kaplan, Kate Gathercole and Claire Gathercole for proofreading, excellent feedback and moral support.
Leon Saponer for the Star of David.
Melanie Grimes for initial stages.
Julian Winston for the Syphilinum dream.
Jenny Taylor for research.
Jenny Malyon for SY.
Sarah Roberts for Hahnemann's Poem.
The publishers of *Fracostoro's Syphilis* for allowing me to publish excerpts:
Fracastoro's Syphilis. Introduction, Text, Translation and Notes by Geoffrey Eatough (ARCA Classical and Medieval Texts, Papers and Monographs 12) Francis Cairns: Liverpool 1984.

And most importantly thanks to Camilla,
who is the inspiration for everything I write.

Contents

For gold the test by fire is made:
True rings the steel of perfect blade:
From poisons healing draughts are riven:
Ships prove their worth when tempest driven:
The soldiers heart's revealed in fight:
The maiden's chastity by night:
While friendship's test will ever be
The touchstone of adversity.

Samuel Hahnemann

Introduction

My aspiration in writing this volume is to amalgamate a number of parallel concepts into a unified and holistic composition that reflects the intrinsic nature of homœopathy.

The first concept is to present a multi-dimensional materia medica. The foundation of this book consists of a description of eleven remedies. To avoid the tedium of long linear dissertations I have presented the remedies in a variety of modes. Each mode has its own lesson and purpose. Some are written as lectures, some as provings or toxicological compilations and others as verse or poems.

In order to wed science and art I have presented original symptoms on one side of the page and remedy portraits on the other. In this way I am hoping to create a whole brain materia medica experience. As each side completes its opposite, it may be difficult to fully understand one side without the other. The pages are colour coded to indicate context and continuity, but feel free to read these complementary sets of data in any order you like.

The poetry was an attempt at delivering my point in a more concise manner, which, for me, turned out to be the longer way by far. Nevertheless I find poetry to be a more refined potency of language, closer to the simple substance of homœopathic expression. The rhythm and metre of a poem succuss the content, while the scant words dilute excessive verbosity. Thus potentised, poetry can penetrate the insulation of bland symptoms, allowing the subtle nature of a remedy to emerge.

Within this diverse structure I have held the principle that all remedy descriptions should be based on fact, meaning rooted in original provings. It is my conviction that in constructing materia medica we must build our castles on firm data, rather than on the shifting sands of ungrounded speculation or insufficient and transient cases. While our imagination soars, our feet should remain firmly on the ground. The original symptoms presented on one side are not merely a copy of the original provings and symptoms, rather a regrouping according to themes. Regrouping symptoms in a variety of configurations will enhance our perception of a proving.

The second concept of this book is the search for an essential principle that unites each remedy. There is more to remedy essences than conglomerations of keynotes, emotions or delusions. Essences should not be confined to mental or emotional portraits, because 'the mind' is only a particular and local reflection of the invisible principle that permeates our entire being. Nor should we let our wings be clipped by the constricting nature of repertory. Beyond the processed language of compiled materia medicas lie original expressions and sensations, and beneath these roots rests a simple core meaning that generates the entire remedy, including physical symptoms. There can only be a single common denominator at the centre of each remedy, a pattern so simple that it precedes all others.

I have concluded each chapter with a synthesis of the remedy, based on a method that I call 'the verb', on which I elaborate later. Much homœopathic effort concentrates on analysing remedies and cases, breaking them down into components. It is important that analysis leads to a synthesis, a concentrated formulation that includes all factors.

The third concept of this book is an investigation of the inner nature of the syphilitic miasm. According to Hahnemann, a miasm is a simple yet powerful disease entity that has infected a large number of people over a long period of time. As a result it creates a huge but meaningful totality, a symptom complex united by a single basic principle. Since a miasm embodies a much larger totality than individual disease, its unifying principle should be much simpler.

The itch of psora is an example of such a simple principle. Seen through the tunnel vision of allopathy, this seemingly insignificant symptom may be perceived as a minor and isolated pathology, yet it has enormous significance when viewed as a symbol of the great psoric miasm. As the most simple symptom of all, it spans the sickness of all humanity.

The search for a basic common denominator of a miasm can be conducted via three homœopathic media – cases, philosophy or materia medica. The study of miasms through cases is difficult, since homœopaths seldom agree on which miasm a particular case belongs to. Furthermore, many cases are complicated by multiple miasms or allopathic suppression. This is especially true for the syphilitic miasm, as it is rare to see unadulterated syphilis these days.

Philosophy may also be a useful tool of inquiry in the search for a simple unifying principle. However, without firm grounding we may drift into fanciful speculation, a common downfall in miasmatic theory.

I have therefore elected to study the materia medica of eleven syphilitic remedies. As the unifying principle of a remedy is the most elementary idea running through the largest totality of its symptoms, we can say that the unifying principle of a miasm is the most elementary idea running through the totality of remedies representing this miasm. Essentially, I am searching for that which is to be cured in the syphilitic miasm by taking the case of it's remedies. In other words, I am attempting to view the miasm 'as if one remedy'. By expanding the concept of synthesis from a single remedy to a group of remedies my aim is to distil the simple principle running through the syphilitic miasm. As mentioned above, this principle would have to be much simpler then the principle of any one of the eleven remedies.

I have chosen archetypal syphilitic remedies, most of which are listed as black type under the rubric 'Syphilis'. In the grimy world of complicated disease, they represent the purest form of miasm available for examination. Two of the remedies, Androctonus and Haliaeetus, have been proved by my Dynamis School. I am publishing my own understanding of these provings for the first time, as ample time and experience have accumulated since the provings.

In expounding the theory of miasms it was not Hahnemann's purpose to create an easy gimmick for finding remedies. Miasms provide us with a map to aid navigation through the chaotic terrain of chronic disease. It is my hope that these writings will advance our search for the key code of this map.

This book is not a compilation of homœopathic data, but rather a guide to homœopathic thinking. I have avoided presenting all my thoughts on a golden platter. As in case studies and pure provings, some of the ideas in this book lie hidden beneath the surface. It is up to you, the reader, to fertilise them by repeated reading and thought.

In this writing lies a part of my soul. I hope it will touch yours.

Jeremy Sherr, 2002

Perceiving Materia Medica

Perception

"...if the physician clearly perceives what is curative in medicines, that is to say in each individual medicine.' (Organon Par 3)

In the quest for perception we seek analogy on every level. Unrestricted by method or memory we utilise the sum of our senses, enhanced by logic, warmed by emotion, illuminated by insight. Finally we distil the totality of our understanding into a single meaningful concept.

Thus equipped we explore the wonders of materia medica. No limiting doctrine, or constricting dogma. No recommended technique or correct mode of inquiry. All that is required is a simple state of being receptive to all potential patterns.

Our search meanders through fields of symptoms, poetic paths, grammatical geometries. Song and symbol, science, riddle, ancient text and modern film weave a web of fact and fancy to mutate musty manuscripts.
And all in the bid for perception.

'The Verb' – Grammar of Pathology

In paragraph 9 of the Organon Hahnemann states that the healthy organism is maintained in dynamic harmony by means of sensation and function. In paragraph 10 he explains that aberrations of sensation and function are the primary manifestations of pathology. It therefore makes sense that in investigating the subtle roots of disease we should meditate on these qualities.

What are sensation and function? From their names we can understand that they are closely related to the nervous system. The nervous system is the most dynamic aspect of human physiology, and as such it is the closest physical manifestation of the dynamic vital force.

Sensation and function are attributes of sensory and motor nerves respectively. This is the body's principal means of maintaining constant homeostasis, the harmony of health. Sensations inform us of any change in the internal or external environment, and functions serve to balance that change with an immediate and efficient response.

If we sense cold, our function is to heat ourselves by increasing blood flow or by trembling. If we sense hunger, our function is to balance by eating or by slowing the metabolism. Sensation and function oppose each other, maintaining a dynamic balance. These operations are circular in nature, and are usually controlled by feedback mechanisms.

The first expression of disease is in distortion of 'sensations and functions'. A person may feel cold in warm weather, or tremble when they do not feel cold. They may feel hungry after eating, or eat when not hungry. Homeostasis is disrupted and ill health ensues.

Sensation and function are a more holistic way of describing pathology than emotions, thoughts or delusions, because they pertain to the whole organism. Pathological sensations are the delusions of the whole person, and functions are the physical, general or emotional response. Experience shows that, the same stuck sensation and function run through all levels of the organism. As such we can use them to find corrolations between physical, mental and emotional realms.

Pathology manifests as stuck sensations and functions, meaning fixed erroneous perceptions resulting in repetitive misplaced response. Or, visa versa, a fixed erroneous action resulting in a perverted sensation. For example, a person may have a continuous erroneous idea that their left side is longer, causing them to lean to the left. Or they may lean to the left due to a perverted function such as scoliosis. The pathological disruption may occur anywhere in the cycle.

The Dynamics of Materia Medica

To study a remedy in the most dynamic way is to prove a remedy. During a proving subtle changes in simple substance ruffle the currents of creation. Prover and remedy are one. No printed word to distort pure experience, no essence or keynote to veil subtle feelings. No longer the intellectual observer standing outside the experience, we become the experience.

A prover is a true student of materia medica. Taught by the subtlest of teachers, the inner nature of a remedy is embossed on her soul, bestowing an understanding finer than words.

A homoeopath who has not participated in a proving has not completed his education. One who has undertaken this alchemical voyage will often be tempted by the next excursion into nature's treasure chest. The knowledge hidden within cannot be gained from books. The process may involve suffering, but the prize is a rich new experience. Care, caution and thorough preparation facilitate a safe voyage.

Provings are a gateway to knowledge. To experience new inner worlds through ones own medicine is a tradition of all shamanic healers. By changing our point of self-reference we gain insight into nature and people. Beyond this personal insight awaits collective wisdom, which lies in sharing the tale. As provers relate their story, a remedy is born. Anecdote and pain, mind and body, eye and soul dissolve to one, enhancing, contrasting, supporting, opposing, completing. Members of the circle experience a feeling of awe as the first ripples of a new remedy spread through the pool of human experience.

But this pure experience must be sifted, printed, sorted and stored. A chronicle is created. As subtle sensations curdle into typeface materia medica spirals down the potencies towards a state of stasis. MM hardens to CM, CM calcifies to 10M. Recorded statements and simple language leave footprints of pure experience, a trail for future generations to study. It is this trail that we must follow while retracing the prover's journey. Pure provings are the foundation upon which the homoeopath constructs his knowledge.

At times it is difficult to tell if the pathology lies in disrupted sensation or disrupted function, as the result (e.g. leaning to the left) is the same. But as a circular mechanism it does not really matter. Sensation leads to function leads to sensation; a snake biting its own tail. We cannot say that one is compensation for the other, because that would suggest that one is the primary cause. It is a 'chicken and egg' situation.

Dynamis means motion, the basis of life. In a state of health we are free to perform any motion at any time, and will choose the appropriate actions in response to accurately sensed situations. Thus we adapt perfectly to change. In pathology we become confined to a fixed sensation or function, true in one particular circumstance, but misplaced in every other situation.

Pathological functions repeat the same actions and are therefore easy to perceive. Grammatically, these symptoms are expressed as verbs. For example, in the symptom 'My green nasal discharge alternated sides', alternate is the verb, discharge is the noun and green is the adjective. The verb 'alternate' is the most dynamic expression of the case, and these dynamic symptoms are often the characteristic. Most strange, rare and peculiar symptoms are verbs rather then nouns, due to their dynamic nature (e.g. Feels hot so he must cover – Camph).

I have therefore called this system of synthesis 'the verb'. It is a description of the constant stuck action in which a person is imprisoned. In health people are free to respond with any possible verb. In pathology they are confined to a single function that indicates loss of freedom. This restricted verb pervades the whole organism. As a stuck repetitive action, people often express this verb as 'must', 'have to', 'should', 'need to' etc. For example, a Silica patient may feel that they 'must push through', both mentally and physically. This is a constant and misplaced function, resulting from a sensation of being blocked, i.e. constipation, suppressed perspiration, delusion he will fail. Every action will express difficulty pushing through against this block (bashful stool, difficult dentition, abscess, splinters, obstinacy etc.) In order to fulfil the constant need to push through, Silica will be compelled to begin the process, retreat and start pushing through again (bashful stool, yielding and obstinate, inserting and expelling splinters, undertaking nothing lest they fail). Thus the function (verb) becomes an ongoing repetitive cycle. This cycle may be perceived in the following symptoms of Silica:

"Sensation as if a bubble of air were pushed through eustachian tube and burst in middle of ear."
"Nosebleed after inserting the finger."
"Obstruction of the nose in the morning, followed by coryza during the after part of the day."
"Difficulty of swallowing; she imagines that she has swallowed pins."

As materia medicas evolve further from their source, original tales stagnate into remedy pictures, poetic symptoms condense to keynotes, verbs harden to nouns. Fantasy lends wings to the armchair voyager. The prover's dynamic expression has been crystallised, calcified and varnished. Clinical cases create new landscapes. Truth and fiction blur as convenience extracts its price.

Yet we would not be without all these. We cannot spend all of our time trekking the proving jungles. Clinical experience, creative thinking, simplification and signatures are all aspects of materia medica. Abbreviation and essences are important aids. Keynotes can point the searcher on his way. All are useful tools of the healing art, but none can approach the precision of a proving. Our healing tools must be accurate, unfolding from proving to case to image, in that order.

In our study of old remedies, we undertake the quest of recreating this dynamic experience, potentising processed material back to original whispers. Retracing the steps of our predecessors, pure proving narrative is our guide. We follow a long gone feeling, seek a line of logic, potentise a pattern. Yet we now possess new tools. Two hundred years of homoeopathic evolution have enriched our perception and enhanced our understanding. Philosophy, analysis, art, science, computer and method have lent power to our inquiry. We may be at the same point in the circle, but we have surely ascended the spiral.

"Language is fossil poetry" Ralph Waldo Emerson

"Materia Medica is fossil provings" J. Sherr

"Silicea taken during the menses seems to suppress them for four days, afterwards they flow for four or five days and then remain away for six weeks."
"He woke with great anxiety about midnight, could not move in spite of every effort, and imagined that thieves were breaking in; on rising he became quiet, after lying down the anxiety returned."

The fixed verb is a constant factor in any proving or case, repeating on every level.
I remember a Silica child who had a repeated pattern of peeking slowly through the door and then hastily retreating. In pathology, a person will tend to excel at performing their main verb, while failing at everything else. Silicas are world champions at the initial stages of pushing through and immediately retreating, but will falter when it comes to going all the way.

Sensations are generally more difficult to perceive then functions, as they demand accurate describing and perceptive listening. They may often be understood from the spontaneous expressions and idioms used in the case, or from dreams. Poor provings and poorly taken cases will not reveal well-defined sensations.

The 'verb' of a case or remedy is its most dynamic expression, equalled only by its invisible counterpart, the sensation. It is interesting to note that certain aboriginal societies have no nouns, only verbs (river being expressed as 'rivering'). As pathology advances it becomes progressively more static, just as all verbs flow into nouns. Nouns (arthritis, tumour, neurosis) are the end result of a pathological process that began dynamically and ended as a fixed entity.

As homœopaths dealing with dynamic forces we should pay much more attention to verbs than to nouns. But we often focus on the more attractive nouns and their adjectives (green discharge, blue monster, hot anger). This is particularly true in dreams. In a dream of a huge black and white dog with purple eyes and yellow teeth jumping over a fence, the jumping is primary, yet many analysts focus primarily on the multicoloured dog.

For example, in the symptom 'My red eruption wanders rapidly', eruption is the noun, the most static and least useful part of the description. Red is its adjective, slightly more dynamic and descriptive. But the most interesting and indicative parts of the symptom are wandering (the verb) and rapid (the adverb), which echo the stuck vital force.

Western physiology and pathology focuses on nouns. In homœopathy, these nouns are termed affinities. Systems of analysis such as the four elements (or Chinese five elements), focus on adjectives – colour, taste, temperature etc. Verbs run silently behind these components, lending them motion and life. From verb to noun is the true progression of hierarchy.

Dynamis

All life moves.
Unfolding, evolving,
soaring and crawling
gently dance to the sun,
it flows.
Growing and shrinking,
constantly seeking
power unseen,
which animates, pushes and
climbs,
it grows.
Vivaciously urging,
coiling and swirling,
pulsating amoebas which breathe,
it swarms.
The moth,
flutters its wings,
leaf curling gently,
salmon leap to the sky,
it seethes.

A soul,
weaving, conceiving,
sensing a meaning,
lovingly answers to sound.
It stirs,
to a verb,
arousing, dictating,
creator creating,
dynamic mutation of nouns,
it speaks,
unthinking, unhindered,
it follows the wind,
and pauses for nothing alone.
Untouched by the stillness
the heart beats its drum,
and sighs,
knowing,
that to stop,

is to die.

In formulating the sensation and function of a case or remedy it is preferable to begin with generals and physicals rather than with mentals. The mind can be a minefield, leading us down the path of speculation.

As an example the remedy Sepia: We can speculate on many mental themes. It would be more accurate to begin from characteristic physical sensations and functions. We recall the Sepia prolapse with a need to cross the legs or hold on with her hands – sensation falling out, function must hold on. We then find the Sepia symptom "Must hold on to something or she will scream". This is a stuck function, something she 'must do'. She has two options, either scream or hold on, i.e. expel forcefully or prevent this expulsion.

We can now scan Sepia to see if there are any other examples of this verb. On the emotional level we recall Sepia's avarice, a need to hold on to money. Looking to the reciprocal sensation, we observe Sepia's great fear of poverty, a fear that the bank account will be empty. We can conclude that it is a fear of emptiness that leads Sepia to hold on so tightly. Thus the consistent sensation is of emptiness. Emptiness of uterus, of bank account, and the well-known description of 'all gone empty sensation' in the stomach. We find the same emptiness in the head, rectum and chest. It is only now that we can understand the true nature of Sepia's emotional state. Drained by child care, menses and stress, she is empty of emotions, to husband, children and life.

To perpetuate the cycle of emptiness and holding on, Sepia must expel, as in scream, prolapse or extravagance. This becomes a cycle of expulsion until empty, then hold on until full. Function leads to sensation leads to function in a circular way. We can summarise the verb of Sepia as 'Must expel till empty, then hold on'. The sensations, driving the functions, are inherent within, i.e. 'feels empty, then full'.

Function and form follow each other. It is interesting to note the form of sepia, the cuttlefish; an empty vessel with tentacles for holding on, forcefully expelling ink. Sensation creates function, function creates form, form begets sensation.

It is not essential to discern exactly which is sensation and which is function. The important thing is that this understanding is not based on speculative analysis of emotions, but on well described physicals and generals. When searching the mentals it is much easier to find the 'verb' of a case or remedy from original idioms. In the Sepia proving we find the following expressions: "She is filled with concern about her health"; "As if he would pine away if he did not kill himself"; "Ideas fly from me"; "Vent my ill-humor"; "Oppressed in sultry weather, but become more cheerful when it thunders and lightens"; "Bloatedness of abdomen... never during walking or dancing". These simple expressions describe the dynamic process of filling

'Philosophy is written in this grand book – I mean the universe – which stands continually open to our gaze, but it cannot be understood unless one first learns to comprehend the language and interpret the characters in which it is written. It is written in the language of mathematics, and its characters are triangles, circles, and other geometrical figures, without which it is humanly impossible to understand a single word of it; without these, one in wandering about is a dark labyrinth.'

Galileo, 1611

and emptying. Later generations of materia medica often become static, losing dynamic verbs to physical or emotional nouns.

Verbs calcify into related nouns, just as the subtle origins of disease result in hard pathology. Naturally it is preferable to perceive and match the whole range of grammatical expression in a single symptom. For example, in the symptom 'He suddenly (adv.) exploded (verb) in hot (adj.) anger (noun), each part of the expression links to its neighbour to form a whole, yet in the dynamic hierarchy, verb is primary to noun. Many remedies are angry, but only some are explosive in character.

Formulating 'the verb' for a remedy or case requires careful and diligent study of original language and provings. It cannot be found by lightly skimming third generation materia medicas or essences. To further illustrate this concept, I have synthesised the sensation and function for each of the eleven remedies.

In my experience, 'the verb' has proved the most useful method for perceiving the essence of remedies and cases, and more importantly, of matching the two. Its power lies in its simplicity and accuracy, in its proximity to the source, and in the fact that it encompasses body and mind.

Organon – Paragraph 16

Our vital force, as a spirit-like dynamis, cannot be attacked and affected by injurious influences on the healthy organism caused by the external inimical forces that disturb the harmonious play of life, otherwise than in a spirit-like (dynamic) way, and in like manner, all such morbid derangements (diseases) cannot be removed from it by the physician in any other way than by the spirit-like (dynamic, virtual) alterative powers of the serviceable medicines acting upon our spirit-like vital force, which perceives them through the medium of the sentient faculty of the nerves everywhere present in the organism, so that it is only by their dynamic action on the vital force that remedies are able to re-establish and do actually re-establish health and vital harmony, after the changes in the health of the patient cognizable by our senses (the totality of the symptoms) have revealed the disease to the carefully observing and investigating physician as fully as was requisite in order to enable him to cure it.

Paragraph 16 Synthesis and Conclusions

Dynamis means 'force in motion'.

The life force is dynamic, i.e. in continuous motion.

The dynamic vital force can only be made sick by dynamic inimical forces, which impede its motion.

Dynamic aspects of diseases can only be influenced by dynamic potencies.

Dynamic symptoms and potencies are sensed and expressed via the nervous system.

The origins of disease are dynamic, while the end results of disease are static. This is homœopathic heirarchy.

Therefore the most dynamic aspects of diseases and remedies are best understood from their most dynamic symptoms.

The most dynamic symptoms are expressed as verbs.

The most static symptoms are expressed as nouns.

Dynamic symptoms tend to be more characteristic.

The more dynamic the symptoms used to match remedy to disease, the more profound the similarity.

The dynamisation of the remedy (choice of potency) should match the dynamic level of the disease. A dymanic homœopath utilises a wide range of potencies.

The homœopath should be in a dynamic state to perceive the most dynamic aspects of the case. Static attitudes perceive only static aspects of cases.

Fracastoro's 'Syphilis'

Fracastoro

The name Syphilis originated from an epic poem written by the Italian physician and poet Girolamo Fracastoro (1483-1553). The poem, "*Syphilis Sive Morbus Gallicus*" ("*Syphilis or Disease of Gauls*," 1530) was acclaimed as a great literary work and an important medical treatise. Among other myths and disease descriptions, the poem recounts the plight of a poor shepherd boy, Syphilis (hog lover). In a moment of rage Syphilis curses Apollo the Sun God, who punishes him by sending him the pox. Physicians in the 1800s chose to call the disease after the poor shepherd's name, Syphilis.

Fracastoro was hailed as the greatest Latin poet of the Renaissance. This was the age of gunpowder, the Reformation, the printed book, the advancement of science and voyages of discovery. It was also an age of terrifying plagues, a time of change in the familiar pattern of disease.

Fracastoro, an important scientist and thinker was involved in some of the exciting events of his age. He investigated the character of contagious fevers and discovered typhus. His theory that infectious diseases are transmitted by invisible seeds of contagion capable of self-reproduction was a precursor of modern bacteriological theories and earned him the title Father of Scientific Epidemiology. He was a dedicated physician, treating the poor for little financial gain. Fracastoro had an extensive knowledge of linguistics and the classics, was a popular man and possessed a fine sense of humour. There have been over one hundred editions of the poem 'Syphilis' with translation into at least six languages.

From Fracastoro's 'Syphilis'

"Syphilus, a shepherd by this very river, so the story goes, used to pasture a thousand oxen and a thousand snow-white sheep over these pastures for king Alcithous: the time was just at the summer solstice; Sirius was scorching the thirst fields, was scorching the groves; and the woods offered no shade to shepherds, the wind offered no relief.

He pitied his flock, and provoked by the fierce heat lifted up his eyes and face to the Sun in its eminence, "Why, Sun, do we call you Father and god of all things and why do we, the ignorant masses, lay out sacred altars and worship you with sacrifice of ox and casket rich in incense, if you have no concern for us and the king's flocks do not touch your heart? Or rather am I to think that you Gods are scorched with envy? By me a thousand cattle, white as snow, are pastured, by me a thousand sheep; you have in heaven, if reports are true, merely one Bull, one Ram—and one dried-up Bitch to guard this enormous herd. What a fool I am, that I don't rather perform divine rites for the king, who has so many estates, so many subjects, whom the broad seas supply and whose power is greater than the Gods and the Sun. The king will grant favouring breezes, he will bring the sweet coolness of green groves to our herds and lighten the burden of the heat." So he spoke; no delay; he set up sacred altars in the mountains to king Alcithous and performed divine rites. This the hosts of country folk followed, this the rest of the shepherd crowd; they burnt offerings of incense at their hearths and they made offerings of bull's blood, and roasted the steaming entrails. When the king heard of this while he happened to be seated on his throne amid a packed crowd of his subject peoples, delighted by the honour due to Gods being shown to him, he decreed that no other godly power should be worshipped on earth, or he would exact punishment; on the world itself nothing was greater than him; the gods lived in the sky, what lay below was not theirs. He had seen these events, who sees all things, who reviews things in detail, the Sun the Father, and he felt indignation in his mind, he hurled his hostile rays and shone with a bitter light. By that glance mother Earth and the sea's flat expanse were attacked, by that venom the air was infected and began to glow hot. Straightway an unknown pollution was born to flood the blasphemous earth.

The first man to display disfiguring sores over his body was Syphilus, who by the shedding of blood instituted divine rites in the king's honour and altars in the mountains sacred to him; he was the first to experience sleepless nights and tortured limbs, and from this first victim the disease derived its name and from him the farmers called the sickness syphilis. and soon the evil plague had spread through all the cities among the commons, nor had it spared in its savagery even the king himself.

...They ask the cause of the evil, what cure exists. She replies: "you, oh, you are being tried by the power of the Sun you despised; with none of the Gods is it right for a mortal to equate himself: give incense to God, and conduct the rites which are his, and appease his power, then he will not carry his anger further. But the plague which he has brought on is eternal and can never now be revoked. Whoever is born on that soil will feel it;

...As soon as she fell silent, the depths of the cave and all the grove shook, and horror stood everywhere around. They executed her commands; they restored to Sun his own altars;

...This sacred tree, which you perceive throughout this grove, which previously had never been known in that soil, immediately began to send green leaves forth from the earth, and to mature in a great forest over the plains. The priest sang that new, annual, rites must be performed to Sun the Avenger without delay. When the lot was drawn it was Syphilus himself who was led away to fall at the altar, one man a sacrifice for all: and now the sacred spelt and the wreaths were ready, he stood on the point of staining the knives with his bright red blood."

From Fracastoro's 'Syphilis'

"... I see a strange, filthy inundation carried through empty space, and great tracts of the sky putrifying. Wars also I descry for unhappy Europe, unholy wars and the fields of Italy running everywhere with blood.

... For a time will come again, by permission of the fates, as the years slip by, when the plague will pass away and lie sleeping deeply in black night; in turn after long centuries that same disease will rise again, and once more visit the heavens and air and again some age to come will regard it with wonder.

... But unusual heat and unusual cold will rise against the world, and the day appointed will show forth new creatures on the earth, cattle and wild beasts will be born spontaneously and take life from their primal source."

Androctonus Amoreuxii Hebraeus

Androctonus – As If One Person

FROM THE PROVING

Increased irritability, a "how dare you!" feeling. Felt like tearing offenders to pieces with his bare hands. He felt an enormous surge of violent emotions at trifles, and had to exercise great control to stop outbursts of violence and impulses to hurt someone. Felt that "everyone were creeps", could not be bothered with anyone. Very strong liking and disliking to people – very intense – ranging from immense sexual attraction to extreme hatred. Spoke with hatred and maliciousness about colleagues. Very sarcastic. Felt angry, did not want to speak to anyone. Extreme mental and physical anguish with restlessness, could not be still for a moment. Assertive, impatient, aggressive. Felt resentful and abused. Had no control over her temper. Bellowed and lashed out at everyone. Wanted to kill her husband and children, banged doors and threw things. I feel afraid of what I might do next. My eyes are staring and full of hate. I have no control over my emotions. Black, horrible moods which don't last long, but are frightening in their violence. In the street, he felt aggressive and very strong, he thought that his umbrella was a knife, and desired to smash people up. Desire to pick an argument or fight. Desire to fight and kill, violent and cruel. It seemed as though he was a different person, very similar to the way he had been in adolescence, but in a much more powerful manner. These emotions were so intense he wanted to rip his chest apart to let them out. He lost all control over his emotions, which seemed to come from a deep and distant part of himself, a darker side. A feeling of great energy and confidence, a magnetic state, his emotions were more intense than ever before. Felt very good in himself, magnetic. Felt very self confident. Self assured, could not care about anyone or anything. My mind is concentrated on one objective and I push aside all distracting influences. A mental tunnel vision. Extremely efficient in his work, did not hesitate. Pushed kids out of bed with no compassion. Things she would normally feel guilt about don't bother her. She was not aware of hurting others' feelings and did not seem to care. Could not appreciate anyone else's feelings. She dreamt that she had murdered her grandfather by poking a knitting needle through his eyes while he slept. She felt no remorse. Increase in sexual power and desire. Sexual desire greatly increased, whole body tense with sexuality, which is purely physical. Sexual desire in presence of any woman. Felt as if would explode with sexuality.

Androctonus Amoreuxii Hebraeus

Evening settles. Orange sun melts into a yellow desert. Craggy rocks, stone and sand form a desolate wilderness, stretching as far as the eye can see. A speckled desert snake, tongue tasting the warm air, has detected its victim. Summoned by keen instincts, a yellow scorpion turns to face her opponent. Now in combat stance, pincers raised, tail arced menacingly, the sharp stinger poises to strike. Defence and attack are one Time compresses into a single instant as a base force takes charge – survive!

Designed to face these moments of danger, scorpions are masters of survival. Their form has proved so successful that they have remained unchanged since moving from sea to land four hundred million years ago. Scorpions can endure extreme conditions and live in almost any climate. They can be found on frozen mountain peaks or in the hottest valleys, and can survive for considerable time without food or water.

Feared by many for their nasty sting, scorpions are formidable fighters. Built like a tank, the tough exoskeleton serves as armour. Strong pincers grasp their prey while the lance-like tail injects its powerful venom. Scorpions are lone warriors, always on guard and ready to attack any potential enemy.

The remedy Androctonus amoreuxii hebraeus was prepared from a small but very virulent yellow scorpion. As may be expected, this remedy exhibits extreme anger and violence. Provers spoke rudely and enjoyed being abusive and sarcastic, reacting with great indignation to the slightest offence. One prover felt an urge to rip people apart with his bare hands. Others stalked the streets in anger, provoking violence. This anger increased into a desire to kill – even their own children. These intense emotions were described as a black thunder bursting from the chest.

In order to survive a scorpion needs to hide. Their normal preference is under rocks or stones. One prover had a desire to put her hands under stones or to hide under rocks. Other cases had dreams of stones or used stones as weapons. This affinity to stones and rocks symbolises the unfeeling and hardhearted attitude of Androctonus.

Feeling of separateness. Felt disconnected from the human race, as if everyone were another species. Totally detached – not from self but from surroundings. I feel entirely alone, that I am viewing the world through one hole, for it all seems just a picture, and the rest of the world share a different view finder together. I don't want to join theirs. She felt separated, detached, disconnected and unreal. Desire to be out in the country, intense desire to be on the rocks. Desire to feel the rocks, to stick hand beneath the rocks, to crawl into or behind rocks. Pains short, sharp, strong, stabbing, poking. Sharp pains in joints of arms, elbows, legs, right hip, knee. Sharp pain in ears, down canal, as if a sharp pencil was pushed down into the ear. Small horny-like growth with spikes on right little toe. Contraction of muscles and tendons. < Evening. < 6–9 pm. Extreme dryness. Skin cracked. Thirst. Aversion to sunlight. Flashes of blue pin points. Strabismus. Retinitis pigmentosa.

Saddam

The dictator Saddam Hussein is a vivid illustration of the Androctonus pathology. He portrays extremes of Scorpion qualities: cold hearted, cruel, cunning and violent. According to biographers, throughout his life he displayed total lack of care for the fate of his fellow human beings. In many instances he was willing to kill so as to get his own way. As a child he beat animals and potential enemies with an iron bar. In 1981 – '82 he ordered the execution of nearly 3,000 people. Eventually he murdered his own family members.

These killings were not the results of a hotheaded rage, as in Stramonium or Belladonna. Rather they were a cold-blooded determination to survive in the world he had created, surrounded by enemies from within and without. In Saddam's paranoid mind every one of his ministers, generals and staff became a potential threat. He showed no remorse or hesitation in murdering them, often personally with a knife. His wife described him as having a heart of stone.

Single-minded determination to fight and win are characteristic of Androctonus. During the Gulf War Hussein never deviated from his goal, regardless of the effects his actions had on family, countrymen, ecology and world opinion. Although he was surrounded by superior armies using the latest laser guided missiles with pinpoint accuracy, he survived. Always one step ahead of his enemies, he directed a masterful campaign from the safety of his underground bunker, hidden deep beneath the desert rock. Scud missiles provided the sting in his tail with which he held his enemies in a state of constant fear. With charismatic magnetism he mesmerised his subjects to following him into a war he could not win, but did survive. Many soldiers from the allied forces have been permanently poisoned by chemicals, vaccinations and fumes.

Imagine innocently picking up a rock, and your surprise at finding an ominous looking scorpion underneath, or even worse, being stung. The first reaction is sudden and intense fear. The fear that is generated by Androctonus is a reflection of the fear they feel, and the anger they display is often based on this fear. Some provers experienced intense fear of being attacked on the street, of driving, dogs or psychic attacks. Another experienced much suspicion and paranoia, trying to outwit friends whom he felt were out to get him.

The Androctonus emotions may characterise adolescents in the stage of alienation and rebellion. They feel like defiant outsiders in a hostile environment. Police, social workers, adults are perceived as the enemy. One prover expressed these emotions as: "I felt like a different person, very similar to when I was an adolescent, but in a much more powerful manner. My emotions were so powerful I wanted to rip my chest open to let them out. These feelings came from a deep and distant part of myself, a darker side." Like Tarentula, there is a sensitivity to music with frenzied dancing lasting all night.

Powerful and charismatic, Androctonus may become a leader of men in times of danger, mesmerizing others with a magnetic personality. Unfeeling and cruel leadership maintains authority, while sharp instinct penetrates the enemies' mind, predicting and intercepting every move.

These Androctonus adrenal attitudes are often fuelled by Hollywood fantasies of lone commandos surviving against the odds by violence and wit. "*Clockwork Orange*", "*Rambo* " and "*Natural Born Killers*", are films that glorify lone warriors. This remedy relishes the intense rush of excitement generated by such movies.

This combative stance often develops in inner cities where conditions of extreme hostility prevail. Police have confiscated packages of 'crack cocaine' stamped with a scorpion emblem. The increase in drug abuse has escalated urban violence and intensified the battle for survival. Staying alive depends on constant alertness, sharp senses and lack of scruples. Jaded drug addicts and dealers torture or kill with no remorse. There is no room for sympathy in their confined reality.

Naturally, not all people living in these circumstances are Androctonus patients. On the contrary, a person living in a seemingly peaceful environment who perceives the world through the narrow perspective of fear and hate is exhibiting a more peculiar and thus deeper state of Androctonus.

The Androctonus behaviour may be excited by betrayal, grief or disappointed love, resulting in a "nobody will do this to me again" attitude. This intensely sexual remedy may

Androctonus Anecdotes

Androctonus has a strong aggravation at 6pm, 6-9pm or twilight. On the circle of four elements this is the area between Earth and Air which is associated with dryness, constriction, yellow, or yellow brown, and the time of approaching death. These are all strong features of Androctonus.

We find much dryness in Androctonus. The skin and mouth are dry, and there is great thirst. These symptoms relate to the yellow colour of this scorpion and its desert habitat.

Constriction and contraction is a general theme, as well as sharp pains. These aspects were typified in the case of a very short 75 year old man who received a dose of Androc. He was in a constant battle with his neighbours. After receiving Androctonus, he reported that his toes, which had been contracted and curled up for his whole life, had uncurled and expanded. As a result he had to buy larger size shoes. He also threw away the glasses he had worn for many years.

The scorpion's need to fight, as well as its toxicology, indicate an effect on the immune system. There have been some positive results with Androctonus in HIV and AIDS cases, which often include an intense sexual component. Recent allopathic trials have experimented with scorpion venom to combat brain tumours.

Astrologically Pluto, Scorpion and Eagle resonate as a trio. Together, these three form a series of the same vibration in various evolutionary phases. The planet Pluto governs the sign of Scorpio, while the god Pluto rules over the shades of the dead in the Underworld. Scorpions are one of the few living creatures to survive in the proximity of nuclear explosions. In ancient times the sign of Scorpio was represented by an eagle. Scorpio must emerge from under the rocks to fight the battle of life, so that the ashes of its ego can transcend into the mighty eagle. In this context it is interesting to compare the remedies Plutonium, Androctonus and Haliaeetus.

react with a series of promiscuous relationships, which they quickly and harshly terminate to avoid being hurt.

Looking beyond the emotional portrait of Androctonus we may focus on the inner nature of this remedy. Like a scorpion's sharp stinger, the central theme of Androctonus is the narrowing into a point. One prover had a desire to attack people with an umbrella, imagining the point was a knife. Another had a dream of sticking knitting needles into the eyes of her grandfather as he slept. For the purpose of survival the Androctonus awareness is concentrated into a single point. This excludes the wider range of 'useless' humane emotions that would impede a battle of life and death. Sympathy and guilt are unnecessary diversions. While other violent remedies may experience sorrow or misgivings, Androctonus has no time for morality. Unfeeling cruelty and lack of remorse are strong features of this remedy.

Another aspect of Androc's constricted consciousness is a sensation of viewing the world through a narrow tunnel or viewfinder. Anyone who does not fit into her point of view belongs to a different species, an enemy to be regarded with suspicion. This gives rise to a sensation of isolation, of being alone in the world and disconnected from the human race. This feeling of separation may extend to a detachment from one's own symptoms, an outsider observing his own condition.

Self-centred and egotistic, the Androctonus world contracts unto itself. Attack is the essence of his being, to be enjoyed with no regrets. Intensely focused on his own survival, he has no concern for the well-being of others. He feels no need to help his fellow man, nor does he desire their favour.

This narrowing theme is also expressed as a highly focused concentration, the ability to focus on one thing to the exclusion of all others. This was described as a 'mental tunnel vision'. Interestingly, there have been reports of scorpion ashes being used to cure retinitis pigmentosa, a disease characterised by tunnel vision.

It is well to remember that, as in all remedies, Androctonus may display a totally opposite state. Like a retired soldier, the unfocused Androctonus may suffer from lack of concentration, disorientation and dullness. Many of the dreams in Androctonus are of being in strange houses, confused. He becomes directionless, clumsy and ineffectual, losing interest in his surroundings. Distant and apathetic, he stares at the window for hours, as time floats slowly by.

As the most intense sign of the zodiac, Scorpios are continually evolving, deeply sensitive, and emotional. They cannot stay stagnant. Their feelings are pronounced with strong attractions or repulsion, deep affections or unforgiving hate. Scorpios are powerful and may use their power for good or for evil. They are known to be tenacious, secretive, capable of deep betrayal and strongly sexual. They are also deeply spiritual. The colour of this sign is a deep dark red.

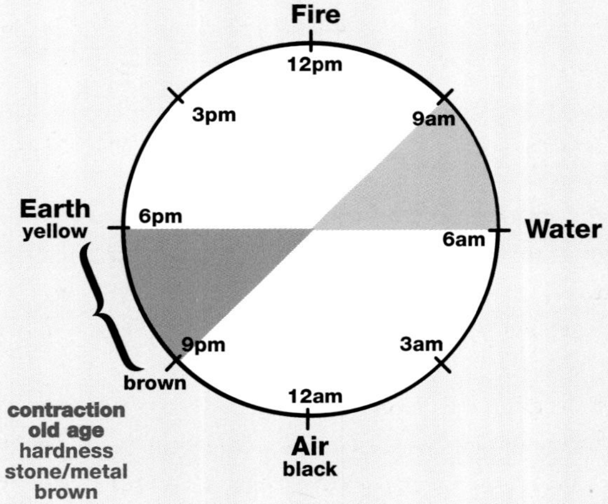

Other Androctonus cases may present as helpless victims of cruel and unfeeling tormentors, who, for 'some unknown reason' are always attracted to them. Under constant attack and abuse, they feel isolated and surrounded. In these cases the prevalent mental pathology is mirrored by the environment. These victims may respond by learning to fight or becoming violent.

It is the sensation of impending violent death that stimulates the Androctonus struggle for survival. Situations of acute fear and danger result in a sudden and rapid constriction of consciousness. These imminent death situations suggest this remedy is in a state of impending transition and transformation. One of my most successful Androctonus cases brought out this aspect. A young man was bought up on a diet of intense abuse and violence, both at home and in school. He was often beaten and bullied, living in a constant state of fearful apprehension. At 11 years old he began intense training in martial arts, in which he achieved many high level black belts. Eventually he became a professional fighter, and could easily handle any violent threat. But the fear remained. He was always on the lookout for the next potential attack. This 'paranoia' began to take its toll physically. His liver and kidneys were painful and he developed vertigo. After a dose of Androctonus he let go of the fear and became much more relaxed, with corresponding physical impovement. He continued to teach martial arts, but in a much softer way, emphasising the 'internal' and spiritual benefits through meditation and self-development.

Just as a warrior must do battle before he can transcend, the scorpion's life or death encounters contain the possibility of transformation. The warrior's ultimate battle is with his own ego, and it's victory lies in the realisation that there is no battle. Hidden within Androctonus are the polarities of sympathy, care for others and the world. The astrological Scorpio is considered the most spiritual of all signs, representing the point of transformation from life through death and into rebirth. Ancient mythology relates the eagle and phoenix to the scorpion. These noble birds symbolise the possibility of transcendence from constricted existence to higher perspectives, a soul soaring to freedom.

There is a point in time in which each of us must summon our inner scorpion and live by the sword, physical or metaphysical. The pathology of scorpion is a state of being permanently stuck in this unique point in time.

Jacob's Ladder

Shadows fall across the plain
dark creeps up the hill,
with a heart as hard
as my pillow stone
and a mind as cold as steel.

It was the last night I would sleep
embraced by my old name,
for if it's called I will reply,
respond, but never feel.

Down the ladder softly
angel of my dreams,
fine as the white
of a moonlit night
light as a moonlight beam.

Via vertex portal
stows into my mind,
laughs, throws back her silver hair,
its you I've come to fight.

I've come to claim
what's left of you,
chill runs down my spine,
why me?
I leap to fighting stance,
you leave no choice, she cries.

Down my ventricle she slides,
eye to eye and mind to mind,
thoughts as fine as sharpest blade,
answer grapples riddle.

Fighting deep in matters grey,
sword to sword and brain to brain
wisdom crushes cunning plans
facts engage enigma.

Battle on
don't let go,
don't give in tonight,
iron jaw, steel resolve
never lose a fight.

Wrestling deftly down my ladder
to thoracic three,
grappling valves of a broken heart,
fight with love says she.

Fierce blow to my midline
seeking refuge at T nine
summon powers deep within
resources of my very being,
the power to continue.

Gasping deep
I throw a punch,
she yields one more time,
blows me down
with a gentle puff
of a hurricane force nine.

Aching bones now yearn to slumber
still we struggle at my lumbar,
pride will not be beat I cry
pride's defeat comes the reply.

Assault to groin attacking knee
hand protecting precious seed,
thrusting forward eager sword
point leaves no impression.

Stars now pale, yield to dawn,
battle rages on and on,
back a step, forward two
using each trick in the book,
up the ladder then she flies
fingers poke between the eyes,
tears surge but boys don't cry
see who fights the meaner.

I curse in the name of my ancestry,
battle moves to lumbar three,
digging feet deep in the ground
searching for my roots, I find,
generation of one plan,
boy to boy and man to man,
fighting for our land, our trees
sacrificing to be free,
youth that never get to be
past the age of twenty three.

'Die' I yell and with a plunge
for her throat a sudden lunge
screaming out my battle cry!
learn to whisper, her reply,
learn to listen to the wind…
at that moment through fatigue
gentle voice slips past my ear,
hint of message faint but clear –
if to win let go your guard,
drop the armour of your heart
let your ancestors depart,
be your truth and learn to soar,
learn to love for evermore.

Deftly parrying my best blow
ducking down and heading low
catches my Achilles heel,
call it ego if you will,
pulls, the pain too much to bear,
bursting up to singe my hair
snake shoots up my spinal ladder
like uncoiling deadly adder,
hot volcanoes, icy shivers,
lightning mixed with fiery rivers,
ecstasy at lumbar one
current surging flaming tongues
rushing up my sacred tree
burning heart gates at T three
bolt of thunder peals high
cuts my voice cervical five,
atlas shrugs and axis ducks
into vertex final plunge
shatters seat of violet crown
bursting out a million suns
up the ladder to the throne
through the sea of all the souls
through the angels wings of gold
to the holiest of goals
silence roaring into my ears,
drowning in a bliss of tears.

Sobbing, dropping to my knees,
Achilles twists right under me,
curling baby on the ground
like a child I hear the sound,
gentle whisper in my ears
singing to my silent tears,
twinkle of her starlit eyes,
telling me I've won the prize,
won the contest of the night,
fought my self and lost the fight,
won the war that has no goal,
faced the darkness of my soul,
still I must continue.

(continued overleaf)

Dynamic Materia Medica, Syphilis

Floating off she melts away,
exhausted I sink in my grave,
feelings speak that have no words,
answers to no question.

It was the last night I would sleep
embraced by rigid truth,
iron spine to soft bamboo,
eyes reflecting youth.

And he dreamed, and behold a ladder set up on the earth, and the top of it reached to heaven; and behold the angels of God ascending and descending on it:
GENESIS 28 :12

And Jacob was left alone; and there wrestled a man with him until the breaking of the day: And when he saw that he prevailed not against him, he touched the hollow of his thigh; and the hollow of Jacob's thigh was out of joint, as he wrestled with him: And he said, Let me go, for the day breaks; And he said, I will not let you go, except you bless me: And he said to him, What is your name? And he said, Jacob: And he said, Your name shall be called no more Jacob, but Israel; for as a prince you have power with God and with men, and have prevailed:
GENESIS 32:25-29

Androctonus Synthesis

Verb

Sensation:
Detached, directionless. Diffused. Unfocused.

Function:
Must contract to a point.
Focus. Viewing the world through a narrow hole.

Noun

Knife, knitting needle, stone.

Image

In a strange house.
Lone alien.
Everyone is an enemy.
Attacked. Threatened.
Must fight to survive.

Intensity. Magnetism. Black thunder within. Hidden sexuality.
Unfeeling cruelty.
Victim of cruelty and multiple attacks.

Related

Anacardium, Apis, Buthus australis, Cocaine, Haliaeetus, Platina, Plutonium, Tarentula
Follows Well: Tarentula
Colour: Yellow, orange, red
Affinity: Nerves, eyes, stomach, rectum, sexual, throat, thyroid, toes, kidney
Time: Twilight, 6pm, 6 – 9pm.

Aurum Metallicum

Corresponding Symptoms

Aurum – Follows well after: Syphilinum(C)
Syphilinum – Follows well after: Aurum (C)
Aurum – Similar action: Haliaeetus, Platina, Syphilinum
Mountain sickness. (Schmidt P.)
Ambition; much, ambitious (C)
Motion: ascending: aggravation (Knerr)
Pain: general: heart: ascending stairs agg. (C)
Very intense, idealistic, want to be the best and set high goals. (Morrison)
Workaholic, industrious; ambition (Vermeulen)
Sadness, despondency, dejection, mental depression, gloom, melancholy: sighing: with (C)
Haughty (C) Audacity (C)
A perfect confusion of ideas. (A)
Mind; Ailments from; love; disappointed, unhappy (C)
Mind; Suicidal disposition; love, from disappointed (C)
Dreams, falling from high places (C)
Succeeds, never (C)
Joy: Death, when thinking of (C)
Melancholy, unfit for world longs for death, which he contemplates with intense delight. (A)
Delusions, imaginations: succeed, that he cannot, does everything wrong: unfit for this world (C)
Despondent melancholy, imagines he cannot succeed in anything (A)
He feels discouraged and despondent; he imagines he does everything wrong and cannot succeed in anything (A)
Delusions, imaginations, fail, everything will (C)
Always disposed to feel anxious for future, even when their prospects are ever so bright. (Teste)
Desires to jump from a height. (Hering)
Pain makes her desperate so that she would like to jump out of window, or dash herself down. (Hering)
Escape, attempts to: window from (C)
Dreams: darkness: being in, all night (C)
Fear: falling, of: heights, from (C)
Motion: descending: amelioration (Knerr)

Aurum Metallicum

Syphilinum climbs
eagle soars
mountain summits
I'll achieve more;

Up, up, up to the sun
striving to climb one more stair
top of the ladder
career and fame
another deep sigh
I'm almost there.

Perfect women
love Platinum men
the essence of falling
is climbing again,

for the kick that I get
at the peak of success
is nothing compared
with the sweet taste of death,

and the time tested way
to sink into pleasure
undertake much
succeed never,

jump from high windows
into dark nights
hitting rock bottom
through fear of heights,

Constant, sulky seriousness and reservedness.(Hahnemann)
Peevish dejection; discontent with all his circumstances; he imagines that he finds everywhere some obstacle in the way; at one time he thinks that this is owing to an unlucky fate, at another that he himself is to blame for it; when the latter was the case he was particularly mortified and dejected. (Hahnemann)
Disposed to fly into a passion. (Hering)
And all the people took off the golden ear rings which were in their ears, and brought them to Aaron…And he received them from their hand, and fashioned with a graving tool a molten calf; and they said, these are your gods, O Israel, which brought you up out of the land of Egypt. (Exodus 32:3 – 4)
The first trituration of Gold was made by Moses out of the remains of the golden calf of the Israelites, and he made the children of Israel drink it in water (Exodus, chap. 32:20). Hence it is also the first Aurum potable on record. (Burnett)
The causes of this state of insanity are prolonged anxiety, unusual responsibility, syphilis and loss of property. (Kent)
Ailments from: Responsibility: Unusual (C)
Cares, worries: full of (C)
Responsibility, duty: strong(C)
Delusions, Imaginations: Neglected: Duty, his (C)
Music ameliorates (C)
Dejected and full of melancholy. (A)
Brooding, melancholy (Kent)
Delusions, imaginations: deserted, forsaken. (C)
Love, unfortunate. (Boenninghausen)
Hopefulness (C)
Grief: financial loss, from (C)
Ailments from: financial loss (C)
Ailments from: business: failure (C)
Mental labor affects him very much; he feels very much exhausted. (Hahnemann)
Memory, impaired. (A)
Prostration of mind, mental exhaustion, brain fag (C)
Reproaches himself (C)
Pining boys; low spirited, lifeless, weak memory. (Boericke)
Feeling of condemnation and utter worthlessness. (Boericke)
Travel, desire to (C)
Melancholia, tedium vitae. (Hering)
Ennui, tedium: entertainment amel. (C)
Suicidal disposition; shooting, by (C)
Suicidal disposition; by hanging (C)

love of dejection
savouring pain
resuming the journey
I'm climbing again,

which way up
what path down
top of Mount Sinai?
Golden calf's crown?

Icarus gliding
too close to the sun
is the pleasure in flying
or taking the plunge,

of duty and burden
which pull to the ground
uplifting music
heart breaking sound,

sweetly forsaken
by lovers long gone
stock market highs
intentions gone wrong,

raising hopes
that let me down
business disasters
mental decline,

condemning myself
above to below
excellent failures
seeking new lows,

excitement of travel
boredom of fun
sniffing more coke
wielding a gun,

Mind; praying (C)
Religious mania, prays all the time. (Hering)
He is all the time imagining that he has neglected something, that he has neglected his friends. He imagines that he deserves reproach in consequence of having neglected duty; he has neglected something, he is wrong, is wholly evil, has sinned away his day of grace, is not worthy of salvation. (Kent)
Proud. (Boenninghausen)
Egotism, self-esteem (C)
Ailments, wounded honor (C)
Contemptuous: self, of (C)
Genitalia, abortion, tendency to (Kent)
Suicidal disposition: abortion, with (C)
Theorizing (C)
Constant rapid questioning without waiting for reply. (Boericke)
The child slept till 3am, then it became wide awake, and spoke in bold tones deliriously, with rapid utterance and red face: "Mother, thou art my gold daughter!" "What kind of dog is that?" "What head is that on the wall?" "What is that running about the room?" and her raving always of questions. (Hahnemann)
"Notice then that peculiar relation between the lungs and the understanding, and between the heart and the will. With every little trouble located in the heart there comes hopelessness, but when the manifestation of disease is in the lungs there is hopefulness." (A general observation in Kent's Aurum lecture, erroneously ascribed to Aurum – JS)
Hatred: revenge and (C)
Object as if divided horizontally so that he can only see lower objects with the inferior half; upper objects remain invisible. (Ward)
Head: half-sightedness, as if upper half of vision were covered with a dark body; sees only half of an object. (A)
In upper dark section of field of vision occasional showers of bright, star-like bodies. (A)
Dreams: Anxious, hemiopia, in (C)
Worse, sunset to sunrise. (Phatak)
The sexual desire, which had been dormant in him for a long time, is roused. (A)
Sexual desire: increased: erections, without (C)
For two nights he is full of lewd fancies, the penis being small and relaxed. (A)
Retraction testes. (Boericke) Atrophy: testes. (C) Undescended testes. (Borland)
As if heart was turning round. (Hering)
Urging in the right abdominal ring as if a hernia… passes off on rising. (Hahnemann)
Head: vertigo when stooping, as if turning in a circle; it goes off on raising the head. (A)
Prolapsus and induration of the uterus. (Hahnemann)
Suicidal with prolapsed uterus (C)

aimed at my head
that hangs from a tree
as my body free falls
I'm down on my knees,

praying to god
salvation and doom
scorn of conceit
glory of gloom,

teacher's gold star
romantic abortion
idealist theories
out of proportion;

Is mother a daughter?
Does hope live in lungs?
Are questions your answers?
Is hatred my love?

Are my eyes hemiopic?
Does vision divide?
Darkness ascending
setting sun rise,

sexual excitement
no rush of blood
testes retract
refuse to make love,

falling upwards
rising down
reversal of fortune
heart turns around,

Throat: ascending into: sensations. (Boenninghausen)
Throat: ascending into: drinks, of. (Boenninghausen)
Arteriosclerosis, high blood pressure. (Boericke)
Violent orgasm, as if the blood were boiling in all the veins (A)
Head, surging of blood to the head with clearly visible carotids and temporal arteries (Vermeulen)
Rush of blood to the head. (A)
Circulation is disturbed: All the blood seems to rush from head to lower limbs. (Phatak)
Coldness of feet seems to ascend to legs. (Medical Advance)
Dreams about dead men. (Hahnemann)
Dreams falling (C)
Contradict, disposition to (C)
Antagonism: herself, with (C)
Delusions, imaginations: heart, turning around is (C)
The general features of the remedy are such as relate to the mind and such as relate to the tissues of the body in general. If you run through the mental symptoms, taking them all in as one great whole, you will see that all the affections, natural to healthy man, are perverted. So great in extent is this that one of the fundamental loves, which is the love of living, of self-protection, is perverted and he loathes life, is weary of life, longs to die and seeks methods to commit suicide. No love of life. (Kent)

abdominal pain
better from rising
uterus descending
blood pressure climbing,

rushing my crown
or surging to legs
joy of despair
dreams of the dead,

while deep below
worthless men mine
for the riches of element
seventy nine.

And all the King's horses
and all the Queen's men
couldn't put
Aurum
the right way again.

But a single dose high
on the tip of the tongue
will turn life side up
and death side down.

Gold Rush

Death death cuddle me,
tantalise seductively,
embracing lovers melt to one,
nurse me to my home.

Death death straddle me,
kiss me with your fantasy,
pluck me from this bed of lies,
take me for your own.

Death death carry me,
comfort me, marry me,
slip your ring unto my finger,
seat me on your throne.

Death define me,
death unite me,
lock me in your milk white thighs,
petrify me,
nullify me,
pluck me from this stark bright life.

Dearest death make love to me,
sanctify profanity,
rock me softly in your arms,
turn my heart to stone.

Wrap me cosy to your breast,
velvet chocolate loving death,
sacred mother tantric lover,
nurse me to my tomb.

Cloak the edges of my life,
in the darkness of your night,
sweet caress me friend of old,
sweet death take me home.

Aurum Synthesis

Verb

Sensation:
Too high, too low.
Heart turns around –
down is up, up is down.

Function:
Must climb up to fall down.

Image

Striving to fail.

Haliaeetus Leucocephalus

Haliaeetus Leucocephalus – Corresponding Symptoms

These quotes represent a small sample of the proving, which should be read in its entirety to gain full understanding of this remedy. The poems are not from the proving.

The Eagle

He clasps the crag with crooked hands;
Close to the sun in lonely lands,
Ring'd with the azure world, he stands.
The wrinkled sea beneath him crawls;
He watches from his mountain walls,
And like a thunderbolt he falls.

Alfred Lord Tennyson

- ***Comparing speeds with others birds.***
- ***Images of being high up and seeing my breast feathers floating on the water.***
- ***I adore the sensation of the wind, of lifting off.***
- ***I feel light, my legs feel springy, the weight on my feet more forward, feel like I am floating around the house.***
- ***Dream: Flying to States for a friend's wedding.***
- ***Kept getting different numbers, like '89th parallel', in my head all day = American.***
- ***Dream, inner vision, memories: Flying north – I could see the straight lines of the Canadian border after I left the Mexican border.***
- ***Inner vision: I was a male Indian. I thought, 'I'm not a brave. I don't deserve this feather.'***

Haliaeetus Leucocephalus

Haliaeetus leucocephalus was prepared from a blood sample taken from an American bald eagle. A year previously, as I strolled the streets of a market fair, I came across this eagle. Right wing and talon injured by a gun, it was confined to lifelong imprisonment and used for educational purposes. Caged, shackled and hooded, it had not lost the commanding air of a king, but had acquired the deep sadness born out of hopeless captivity.

Naturally, it is quite difficult (and illegal) to obtain samples of a free and healthy eagle. Haliaeetus reflects the predicament of this specific eagle, which befits its use in analogous situations. Its proving contains aspects of animal, blood and tragic personal history. As with any remedy, when prescribing according to a particular proving, one should use remedies derived from the original potencies.

This proving created an unintentional experiment. The brave provers of Haliaeetus had actually volunteered to prove a radioactive remedy, and were under the impression that this was the case. Yet the proving contained no speculative reference to radioactive phenomena. The undeniable similarity of the remedy picture to the signature of this particular eagle and its unfortunate personal history serves as a powerful validation of the proving process.

Undoubtedly, the inner nature of eagle is conveyed through the proving. Sensations of flying though the air or above the clouds. Visions of birds soaring together, talons locked, plummeting in exhilaration through whooshing winds. Dreams of flying over barren terrain looking for a new home. Elevated and hollow sensation in the bones, wanting to walk with arms outstretched. Thoughts of Superman or Icarus. Even the leucocephalic nature of the American bald eagle manifests as an attraction to men with white hair. The name bald is erroneously derived from 'blanc', the French word for white.

The American bald eagle is native to North America and a symbol of the United States of America, a theme that arises in the proving. Images of flying over the parallel lines of the Mexican and Canadian borders, dreams of Native Americans, or of walking over old maps of the USA. Although the eagle was revered and considered sacred by many native cultures, it was despised as a scavenger by Benjamin Franklin and hunted by Europeans and white Americans.

- *Deep depression. Have sunk as low as I can.*
- *I hit bottom and bounced back up again. Feel as low as I was high. Reached a low point. My bounce is gone. I felt pathetic, defeated and vulnerable. Enthusiasm is down. Low outlook.*
- *Am thinking about taking a job that would put me in a high class, but don't know if I would want to work with those kind of people.*
- *Good spirits. I feel grounded and centred today.*
- *Feeling ungrounded and out of body; walking but not seeing, aimless, without a mind of my own.*
- *Don't feel I have any direction. Usually I have a direction though I might not know where it is going to lead. Now I feel lost, like I have no ground under me. I have no idea.*
- *It felt like I was in prison or the thing in me was in prison.*
- *Intense trapped feeling. I felt trapped by people and situations.*
- *Like a caged animal, snarling. I'm in a pressure cooker.*
- *Despair and frustration, like a group of ragtag Indians who have been confined to a reservation and can find no glimmer of hope, no way out.*
- *I feel desperate. We're a rag-tag group without luck, or leadership, fighting a losing battle.*
- *Overwhelming gratitude that I can walk and am not confined to a wheelchair.*
- *My arm feels like a broken wing.*
- *Dream I got an escort to my car. Then we were both shot and paralyzed.*
- *Feel self-destructive, like eating greasy fatty junk food, not exercising, slowly kill myself that way. Why care?*
- *Part of me that wants to disintegrate and die.*
- *I was feeling very self-destructive. I wanted to do crappy things to myself. The border's breaking loose. Screw it all, the futility of it all; the futility of working toward the positive, of caring for my health, of doing good things. What for?*
- *It's all about feeding and flying.*
- *A sensation as if some danger was near.*
- *Sense of danger; being just around the corner.*
- *On the way home, I smelled a wood fire and I thought right away that my house must be burning.*
- *In shock about missing court filing deadline. Paralyzed about what to do. Mixes up words when talking. Drifting off. Unable to hold a train of thought. It's like fighting an enemy you can't see that keeps hitting you from behind.*
- *Looking for an escape. Started calling airlines to see when and how I could get away.*
- *Pictures of the mountains make me homesick. Deeper than homesick. Feeling low, remembering the freedom of going to them. Missing mountains and the outdoors.*

The emotional configuration of Haliaeetus is unique. Although it is composed of elements common to many other remedies, the totality forms a singular entity that has no parallel in the materia medica. I recall the proving of Haliaeetus as being an intense and occasionally disturbing experience. Psychologically, this remedy is characterised by extreme emotions, ranging from euphoria to deep depression and despair. The elation is expressed by "up" words, obviously related to the eagle's capacity to fly higher then almost any other living being. *"High," "uplifted," "elated" "bouncy," "jubilant,"* and *"jumping for joy"* were used to describe feelings of confidence, contentment and ease. Provers were able to come to quick decisions and relate to others in a direct and straightforward manner. The upward motion was also expressed by a concern about social and financial position, a desire to ascend to a higher social class.

Another expression of the eagle's nature are sensations of being grounded or ungrounded. The feeling of being in solid contact with the ground is associated with stability and calmness, while the ungrounded sensation is associated with airiness, aimlessness, and lack of direction. This loss of direction is in opposition with the eagles amazing navigational skills, and may be expressed as irresolution, confusion of identity or a feeling of having no goals.

At the opposite extreme of elation, Haliaeetus can experience profound and deep despair, lack of motivation, frustration and low self-esteem. This remedy reflects the sad predicament of our eagle as a lifelong prisoner. Like a caged bird with clipped wings, provers experienced total helplessness and dejection, together with despair of ever escaping their miserable plight. The wounded history of this eagle is also expressed through dreams of being shot and paralysed or sensations of being blasted by a thunderbolt. One prover had powerful memories of an old injury where she was told she would never walk again. Thus we should consider Haliaeetus in 'no hope' or 'endless' circumstances resulting in despondency and desperation. Life imprisonment, being maimed or profound grief are situations that come to mind. The plight of the Native American's people, confined to reservations, is a interesting analogy to this eagle's predicament.

> *"Feels like we're the American Indians. 'Here's 24 dollars worth of beads for your island, idiot.' In the pit of despair."*

As a result of this intense and hopeless despondency, the Haliaeetus condition may deteriorate into self-destruction. There is a desire to disintegrate, avoid exercise or eat unhealthy food. Provers attempted to overcome the 'groundless' feeling by constant eating, which, coupled with the self-destructive tendencies, may indicate this remedy in eating disorders. Sensations of being fat or ugly were associated with desire for fatty food.

- *Want to get in the car and drive forever.*
- *Feel like a rushing train. Like diving from a high dive and there is no water in the pool.*
- *Aggravated driving to work. Why don't these people get out of my way?*
- *I'm coming across with too much force. I find myself shouting at everyone much more than usual. Like a crazy person. Impatient over others' slowness.*
- *Intensely irritable, annoyed at every little thing; a complete bitch.*
- *It's been a long time since I've felt this angry. Children are an obstacle to enlightenment.*
- *I have to kill the children. They are not obeying me.*
- *Wanting to hurt, to be cruel. Wielding or throwing a knife.*
- *I want to kill or hurt someone, and I would have no regrets if I did.*
- *While I was in the shower, I just wanted to kill.*
- *While playing with a small puppy, desire to crush its head, to experience the sensual enjoyment of tearing flesh from bone. A strong feeling of power over the helplessness of smaller creatures.*
- *My vision is focused and sharp, seeing long distances clearly.*
- *I can see forever, see individual midges at 50 yards.*
- *Feel clear and focused, I can put things together clearly.*

Hannibal Lecter

In its extreme, the pathology of HAliaeetus LEucocephalus is typified by HAnnibal LEcter, antihero of the movie "Silence of the Lambs". An insane and cruel criminal, he took great pleasure in killing his victims, and was destined to spend the rest of his life in a cage. Although his intense focus instilled great fear in all around him, he also projected a majestic quality and an affinity to raw justice.

- *I could see where I am going in a long term time frame, versus just short term goals.*
- *Eyes feel nearsighted. Don't want to look far away. Don't want to go far out of my house either, not even to the market. Don't want to go far outside my territory. On an inward adventure. It's like my eyes only seeing close, and not far away.*
- *My eyes have soft focus, like walking around in a fog and thinking in my head.*
- *It takes more effort to focus eyes. Eyes feel tired. I want to stare off out the window.*
- *Must pull myself back to focus to read. Focus is hazy and soft. Letters look jumbled, out of focus. Similar to my mind. Can't focus and have no desire, no motivation or ambition to do it.*

Nourishment and food are an important part of this remedy, especially issues of feeding the young. Like some other bird remedies, Haliaeetus may have intense desire or aversion to eggs. Other foods symptoms were desire for fish, especially salmon, and aversion to sweets, chocolate and cooked food.

Haliaeetus experiences intense anxiety and suicidal thoughts. Fears centre around a sense of impending danger, imagining that something bad is about to happen. Fears that her house is burning, of floods, of cancer and of death. A sense of shock from any adversity. Strong desire to escape resulting from a feeling of being boxed in. Homesickness with a yearning to be free outdoors, especially in the mountains.

The least disturbance results in irritability and impatience. This impatience is especially aggravated by any impediment of flow. Impatient with slow traffic or with a shopping trolley in the supermarket. Desire to drive fast and exhilaration at the sense of flowing speed. He feels as on a roller coaster or a rushing train, and is frustrated by any obstruction. *"I am in hyperdrive."* These urges are contrasted by an opposite sense of inertia and lethargy, an inability to start things or to get going. *"Everything is in slow motion and I can't contact reality."*

The anger of Haliaeetus is intense. Easily insulted with no patience for others. Annoyed at people talking and aversion to company and conversation. Blaming others, critical, shouting at the children. A feeling of being right and desire to enforce her ideas with little consideration to others opinions. In its most extreme state, this anger can develop into violence and desire to kill. Threatening to kill the children for any disobedience. One prover delighted in imagining how it would feel to crush a small puppy while another wanted to kill and eat a rabbit raw. There is no guilt or morality accompanying these impulses, an uncaring and remorseless attitude. Haliaeetus may take pleasure in its violence, and could fit the profile of a serial killer.

Obviously the emotional profile of Haliaeetus reflects many of the eagle's characteristics. Yet we can rise above the limited and essentially 'sameopathic' view of 'Eagle picture equals Eagle remedy.' Although this approach may yield results, similitude echoes many levels of analogy. By focusing our inner vision, we can perceive deeper parallels to bridge the chasm that splits nature from its reflected human suffering.

A close study of the symptoms reveals a powerful affect on the eyes and vision. Sight is the bald eagle's most important sense, and its distance vision exceeds ours fourfold. While the human retina contains one depression called a fovea, the bald eagle's retina contains two, creating vision that is both sharper and more powerful than ours. This remedy has a

- *Can't focus on the larger wide and philosophical goals, on the big picture.*
- *Seeing color in the sky. One time it actually did turn into two faint rainbows. Wonder if I'm noticing a larger spectrum of light and seeing it before it actually happens.*
- *I know the time exactly without looking at the clock. I know my position in time and space.*

> *They don't look at us;*
> *they see into us!*
> *An eagle's stare*
> *from an icy sky*
> *or bare bough*
> *pierces like a laser.*
>
> *The mystery-dark circles*
> *centered in the yellow iris*
> *of his eyes*
> *focus keenly.*
>
> *Visionary power concentrated,*
> *they have, indeed, penetrated*
> *the center of man's being.*
>
> White Deer of Autumn

- *Remembering the spray region of the atmosphere which is below the magnetosphere and above the ionosphere in the exosphere. Ionisation. Magnetism occurring with sunspots.*
- *Horizontal magnetic forces. The sun's gravitational attraction.*
- *Pictures of sun-spots in parallel lines. That made me laugh – the fact that they were parallel.*
- *I feel I'm held together by the bridge of my nose.*
- *My eyes feel different looking out – they feel wide again.*
- *Seeing faces – these were human faces, broadened in the middle with the eyes round to the sides. They changed from human to birds to fish.*
- *Got excited – beautiful parallel lines in the sky – I felt elated.*
- *Parallel universes. Maybe I was in a parallel universe and its all happening the same somewhere else.*
- *Inner vision: like travelling in space – lots of movement past stars, mainly in the space between the parallel lines of the Milky Way.*
- *I bought 12 duvet covers – 6 of them have parallel stripes.*
- *Pain with onset of menses, shooting down from uterus to hips then down inner thighs, like twin straight parallel lines pulling on either side of the pubic area, down thighs to knees.*
- *Inability to reconcile different points of view. A feeling of being pulled in two different directions by two powerful elephants.*
- *Spine feels as if it is in two pieces at the lumbar-sacral junction, like an earthquake fault-line. Feels as if two things aren't lining up right.*

strange sensation that the eyes are balls rolling around in the sockets. There is an increased sensitivity to the whole spectrum of light waves, as if the eyes were satellite dishes, receptors for microwaves or stellar signals. Sensation as if the eyes were wide open and able to take in a lot of light. Seeing rainbows, sunspots, deep purple colours, white light or full spectrums, wavy motions of air, showers of molecules. In spite of this sensitivity there is an ability to gaze directly at the sun. Haliaeetus' extreme clarity of vision is mental as well as physical, at times 'seeing' things clearly before they happen.

Bald eagles are sensitive to the magnetic fields of the earth. It is believed that eagles can calibrate light from the sun with magnetic forces and use this information as a compass during migration.

Associated with this visual acuity are polarities of focused or unfocused vision, a key to the remedy's nature. There may be extreme inability to focus the eyes and difficulty with accommodation at varying distances. In one instance a prover's eyes were unable to function in unison, as if trained in two different directions.

These strange phenomena may relate to the eagle's anatomy. Due to the position of the eyes on both sides of the head, separated by the great beak, there may be double or parallel vision, with an ability to focus only at long distances. Both eyes face forward, giving the eagle binocular vision which allows for the precise depth of field necessary when diving from the sky to snatch prey. Unlike human eyes, the eagle's eyes are autonomous, allowing independent monocular vision to the sides. A peculiar symptom related to this phenomenon in this regard was:

> *"When I tip the book at an angle the typed lines go into a 'V'. The book has to be straight horizontally, if tipped the lines become a 'V' down the centre of my field of vision and I can't read."*

One prover regained depth perception (dependent on the stereophonic use of both eyes), which had been lost following a head injury 30 years previously. This lack of focus and the independent function of the eyes reflect an inability to converge to a point, like two lines that never meet. It is here that the theme of parallel lines in the remedy becomes apparent.

"Noticing more lines – parallels."

"The thing about parallel lines is they never come together. I was drawing parallel lines and they never met."

- *Back feels split as if two planes are pulled apart, like after an earthquake.*
- *Crack in centre lower lip.*
- *Occipital headache parietals – bilateral.*
- *Split in the line of vision.*
- *I was flying and could see lots of lines on the land. Some were parallel. Some were natural and some were like railway lines. Railway lines across the continent.*
- *It feels as if everyone is on rails.*
- *With the sound of a passing car outside saw and heard the sound of a railroad, the first train travelling across the USA from east to west. I was above looking down.*
- *Dream: I was travelling on a train.*
- *Dream: I was being told all the answers to the parallel lines…The parallels were to do with horizontal magnetic lines, tracks and the poles. These were the signposts on the land and are what you follow, the poles, measurements, far horizons, and the importance of the East.*
- *As the sun rose over my house, felt there should be two suns. Desire for symmetry in the sky.*
- *Feel lopsided with just one sun – I lean over to the right.*
- *After I looked at the sun, I saw an inner vision 4 suns in a ring connected to each other and to another one above with strings of light.*
- *There's still only one sun. There was a space over to the right when it was rising where there should have been another one. Then it was central and it was OK. And then when it was higher and had moved over to the right, the left side had an empty space. There should have been two suns. The sun has now changed angle in the sky and rises central to my vision. Better. I am able to gaze directly into the sun.*
- *I also keep hearing the word 'parallax' – its a word used in astronomy that is something to do with how I see the sun in the morning. I can actually look into the sun – this relates to parallax.*
- *I also felt like I should be outside, but there wasn't a sun or stars, so what was there.*
- *Felt strange not seeing the sun the last few days. I can't get my bearings.*
- *It felt like I was on the edge of a psychotic break. Like I could just go crazy and completely lose it. A lot of agitation and irritability on the surface. Underneath there was a crevice, a crack... in my soul or the universe. I would describe it as a painful, frightening, and uncomfortable negative spiritual experience.*
- *Fear of approaching insanity, of going crazy.*
- *During the proving all the bits and pieces that seemingly had unique personalities of their own were simply more broken up.*
- *Sad that there is a crack, a possibility my relationship might end.*
- *Relationship with husband disintegrating.*

"I am parallel to myself, dual, but not divided."
The image of parallel lines also manifests in a significant theme of railway tracks and trains. It is possible that the eagle uses these tracks as a landmark while flying over the vast, featureless terrain.

Side by side with the theme of parallel lines is the peculiar notion of two suns. It seems that the eagle's parallel vision and great receptivity to light produce, in the proving, an ability to see an extra sun or image of a sun that humans cannot perceive. The eagle's ability to perceive two suns may serve as a navigational aid by enabling it to calculate the distance and position of the suns at a given time. A prover explained that the only time there should be one sun was at noon.

We should now focus on the characteristics that result from this parallel configuration. In this regard, Haliaeetus' closest analogue is Syphilinum, which shares the parallelism and its opposite, convergence to a point. These two remedies share self-destructive tendencies and a feeling of never-ending torment. As expressed by a prover, parallel lines can never meet. *"Something has started and I don't know where the end is. It's an endless feeling."* Thus Haliaeetus, a remedy made from blood, most probably belongs to the syphilitic miasm.

One factor that differentiates Haliaeetus from Syphilinum is that it focuses not on the lines, but on the eternal split between them.

> *"It's like a deep, deep crack and it is getting deeper, like a crack in my soul. The crack has an endless quality to it, like a crack in my soul or the universe. It feels as if the gates between conscious and unconscious are opening, as if the gates of hell are open. Extreme power of darkness. Life seems like hell, a negative spiritual experience, painful and frightening. All the beauty and order are gone. Horror of the extreme evil force of darkness emanates out of this crack, reminding me of extermination camps and killing machines. Is that where Hitler came from? The crack in the universe? I would like to fling that vial of remedy to the end of the universe."*

As well as being the symbol of the United States, Rome and Russia, the eagle was a symbol of the Third Reich. The frightening and evil sensations led to desperate praying in an attempt to ward off the unending horror of a cracked parallel universe.

> *"I read prayers for safety before bed because I was afraid of what might happen when I went to sleep. When I came to the phrase 'God is One', I realised that was the crux of it – the universe was cracked or split instead of one. Saying that prayer feels healing."*

- *Got really angry with my partner. I wanted to shake her. Something in me was evil, taking over me and I could not tell her. This is not me. She saw it as me. I was very sad about that. She still doesn't understand. That has been a hard thing for me. Our relationship broke up during the proving. I found there was great freedom in being real, instead of playing around in the romantic phase. She had difficulty in being grounded. I'm a very grounded person, difficult for me to be an airy fairy flighty kind of person.*
- *Why am I mostly on my own? I'm not lonely with so much beauty but desire a mate – a parallel – together but still space in between.*
- *On a high, synchronistic. Almost too overwhelming. I'm one with the universe.*
- *Feeling relaxed and in the moment, in the right place at the right time; a sense of well-being and relaxation.*
- *I'm suspended, doing nothing, just sitting and staring. No chatter, just silence, totally present and quiet. One with the space.*
- *It was as if there was no history between us (me and husband), relating more in the moment.*
- *In the middle centre of the brain – pleasure centre activated.*
- *Definitely much calmer. Feel very alert, present, calm and relaxed, no mind talk that I usually have. Remain calm with external stress.*
- *I get energy rushes like from a good meditation or a martial arts workout. I felt in the moment. Every moment is an eternity.*
- *I feel really calm like when you look at a sunset. It's just there. A deep peace.*
- *I feel so much more present and relaxed in life. The word witness comes up.*
  That playing the game, giving in to evil, isn't an option, and playing to beat the game, hoping to beat the structure while still a part of it, won't work either. So where does one take appropriate action? I see a big crowd of people, one by one withdrawing themselves saying, 'I'm not going to play that game anymore.' Being 'still' in the face of passion, anger, fear and righteousness. Not even passive resistance, but turning the mirror of witness on the game so the participants can see what they are doing and drop their weapons.
- *Good guys and bad guys. Drama of evil is set up by the bad guys. They always win, always a struggle to just keep going. During the proving, I saw that even engaging in that struggle gives it power and meaning. If you stop and watch the game, eventually there won't be anyone playing anymore.*
- *At the same time being outside looking at it all, watching, objective, and seeing the big picture. Distancing.*
- *I felt as if the good things were like a mirror to the other side.*
- *Even more tolerant at opposition or differences of opinion.*

The intensity of this crack in perception may lead to the edge of a psychotic breakdown. Life becomes perpetual, meaningless and repetitive. Trying to keep busy to negate the horror of an eternal abyss.

> *"I felt like I could just keep eating eggs; fry an egg and eat it, fry an egg and eat it, fry an egg and eat it. An endless frying and eating of eggs. Everything is so meaningless, like you could lie in bed forever, or eat eggs forever."*

This endless parallel torment may result in maniacal behaviour, anger, speediness, and euphoria. In extreme states this could progress to fragmentation of the personality.

> *"I can't stand it any longer. Feel on the edge, the borders are breaking loose, I'm going mad. Spiralled and spiralled. There's no escaping out of this. In a total frenzy, like steaming horses that have escaped, running down the road. Experienced many fragmented personalities, all changing in rapid succession. Feel like a rushing train, like diving from high, but there is no water in the pool."*

> *"Fragmentation is the denial of will. Integration is the use of will. All separate states under a unified country."*

Relationships crack and disintegrate, often due to self-sabotage, an urge to destroy. Fighting with partners, husbands, wives. Feeling of a glass wall separating mother and child. Yet Haliaeetus is also capable of feeling intense sympathy.

> *"Feeling for people, puppies and just feel my heart. I was more empathic, feeling other people's pain, almost to the point of weeping."*

It is apparent that this remedy may be suited to intense situations. Some of the provers experienced profound suffering. Soaring and plummeting the extremes of an eagle's experience is not an easy journey, yet the exalted flight and vision offers a great compensation. As the eagle ascends the height of awareness, divergence meets at a single point of consciousness. Past and future unite into the present and time melts into oneness.

> *"It seems as if the past and the future have collapsed into the present. The past was unimportant, and I don't concern myself over the future."*

> *"I'm in the moment. Every moment is an eternity. Who is writing this anyway? Everything is so still. Everything has stopped."*

- ***I now actually enjoy listening to people express opinions I don't necessarily agree with. I continue to feel calm, able to listen, and not get caught up in the fray.***
- ***Where is the truth and justice they talk about? Why do humans lie and deceive? I feel a big thing about truth and justice – Why don't these people just tell me the truth? It feels like a game, not telling me what they really want and need.***

Relationships

The sun is an important feature in Haliaeetus. Provers felt there should be two suns in the sky, or felt very lost when the sun was hidden. On a general level there is burning and radiating heat. In this context it is interesting to compare Haliaeetus to Helium. In addition to the similarity in name, Helium is the symbol of the sun and a result of nuclear fusion. The proving of Helium has interesting similarities to Haliaeetus, such as clarity, a desire to be alone in the mountains and floating sensations. Even more remarkable in Helium is the peculiar delusion of being an eagle. Just as Helium is a noble gas that floats to the top of the atmosphere, so is the eagle noble king of the skies.

There is an ancient mythological triad consisting of scorpion, Pluto and eagle. Haliaeetus has many similarities to Androctonus, sharing the scorpion's intense focus, as well as its cruel, uncaring and violent disposition. Eagle's capacity to observe from above corresponds to Plutonium. If we combine the remorseless aggression of Androctonus with 'the observer from above' of Plutonium, we approximate some of the attributes of Haliaeetus.

The result of this presence within the centre of time is a state of deep contentment and harmony. Tranquillity is a symptom common to a number of remedies, and can be difficult to use in a clinical setting. However, the tranquillity of Eagle leads to a unique characteristic. This is a state of witnessing, a pure objectivity that will not take sides in the worldly struggle of parallel and opposing teams that can never share a common point of view. Aloof in its elevated awareness, Haliaeetus detaches from the human folly that revolves around eternal strife.

> *"It is the structure that people who are bad within the structure fight the bad. The only way to do anything is to sit back and witness the set up, not be a part of the structure for either good or bad. People as individuals are pulling out of the game of good and bad. It's a bad people's game and you can't win. Playing it just supports the game, even if you are one of the good people. Good people get co-opted into being just as bad as the bad people. What is right action? The drama was clear; the good guys and bad guys. During the proving, I realised it all leads to the same thing. Withdraw. Acting/watching. A chosen separation. Zen state of watching and witnessing."*

From this highly objective position eagle approaches the state of a truly unprejudiced observer. We may postulate that at its core the noble eagle retains a 'pre-psoric' stance and is therefore an antipsoric as well as an antisyphilitic.

The Kabala teaches that the Tree of Life is constructed of three parallel columns. On the left side is the pole of Judgement and discrimination, and on the right side is the pole of Sympathy and benevolence. Haliaeetus separates these polarities to an extreme degree. But, in opposition to the deep and evil crack mentioned earlier, it also has the power to unite both columns in the central column of Mercy, which represents divine presence.

> *"To have caring, there must be an attunement with the oneness of the universe. Oneness is about caring; the split is about not caring."*

Though the internal configuration of Haliaeetus is the unfocused separation of parallel lines, which leads to a dark, empty abyss, in our vast curved universe parallel lines may eventually meet, high above the ground or deep within our interior. Once the eagle focuses on this central point of view, it can align with the only force in the universe that is beyond good and bad, present and future, judgement and sympathy – the all powerful force of God's light.

> *"Inner vision. I was sunning my wings in the dawn sun – I'm not flapping –soaring – not dusk, at dawn – not for dark, of Light."*

Doth the eagle mount up at thy command, and make her nest on high?
She dwelleth and abideth on the rock, upon the crag of the rock, and the strong place.
From thence she seeketh the prey, and her eyes behold afar off.
Her young ones also suck up blood: and where the slain are, there is she.

Book of Job 39:27-30

"Woke with a funny dream – it was a bit like Superman – I was a writer for the 'Sun' newspaper and my title was 'Forces of Light'. I was really working for the Sun, a large dark bird, with the 'Forces of Light'."

Haliaeetus leucocephalus is a complex remedy, containing many diverse aspects. Its range of action spans deep despair and timeless elation, cruel aggression and harsh justice, parallel schisms and focused unity. But beyond the complexity lies a singular concept, of which the following quote is characteristic:

> *"Trying to get things organised at home, which is like trying to get my eyes focused. Other times I just stared out the window, unfocused. When I'm unfocused, it's like a place where you can get lost, as if you're going to lose it. Unfocused is like going into the abyss, from which I won't come back, go crazy. I either feel totally in flow with the universe, or floating aimlessly down a river. When I'm focused, I bring it all in, in the present, there, like meditating, or seeing God. God is One."*

Haliaeetus

Five thousand feet above the earth an eagle soars. Wings spread in majestic span, freedom rides a thermal, white mane trailing a crown.Unfocused gaze defies the two suns, royalty surveying its kingdom.

Far below, miniature human ants struggle on; nose to ground, bumper to bumper, lawyer to lawyer. Black army stabbing white morality, white army fuelling black flame. Traversing the great plains, railway tracks stretch on forever like latitudes on a map.

Aloof, aloft, eagle flies the moment, refusing affiliation.

Suddenly, a rabbit moves. High above, keen eyes focus, rushes of adrenalin hunt the pleasure of kill. Eagle dives, hurtling towards its prey like a thunderbolt from the sky. Three thousand feet, then two, now one, death's smell intoxicating senses as claws shred flesh from bone. Then, lifting its victim a powerful flap of wings propels upwards, seeking the safety of sky.

A shot rings out.
Searing pain, spiral dive.
Reality cracks, splitting the world.

Gateway to insanity.

Haliaeetus Leucocephalus Synthesis

Verb

Sensation:
Split in two directions.
Deep crack between parallel worlds.
Unfocused.
High and low.

Function:
Must focus into one.

Image

Split world; insanity. Hyperdrive.
High and low – Grounded and ungrounded.
Endless despair of captivity. Indian reservation. Self destruction.
Cruelty, knife.
Detached oneness. Unprejudiced observer.

Guaiacum

Guaiacum Analysis

The Tree: Lignum Sanctum, Lignum Vitae

- Guaiacum is an evergreen tree; the stem is almost always crooked; the wood is extraordinarily heavy, solid and dense, hard and durable, and is mainly used for doorknobs, hinges, spindles, gear-wheels and sheaves (affinity to joints).
- Used to make police truncheons/batons.

Contraction

- On waking in the morning, everything seems too tight.
- Muscles and tendons are contracted resulting in painful rigidity and swelling of the joints.
- Muscles seem too short - eyelids, back, thigh etc.
- Short tendons.
- Contractions between scapulae; palms etc.
- Toothache on biting them together.
- Constrictive sensation in the region of the stomach, with anxiety and difficult breathing.
- Dull griping in the lower abdomen.
- Tension in the thighs, especially in the right, as if the muscles were too short.
- Painless constriction in the right calf.
- Progressive emaciation.
- Emaciation and hectic fever.
- Arthritis of the wrists, ankles and knees.

Stitch/Ending in a Stitch

- Violent large stitches in the brain from below upward.
- Dull pressive pain in the head, which ends in a sharp stitch in the right frontal eminence.
- Dull pressive pain in the head, extending obliquely upward from the left side of the neck to the vertex, ending in a stitch.
- Dull drawing stitches, extending from the left parietal bone to the frontal eminences, where they all end in a single stitch.
- A pressive drawing-tearing stitch in the right side of the head, extending toward the frontal bone.

Guaiacum – Tree of Life

Deep in jungle
land of sun
grows a sacred tree,
to sail the seas
and heal the curse
of the divine
disease.

Tree contracted
convoluted
growing very slowly,
turns and twists
like condensed metal
sinks in water,
stony.

Old world new world,
east meets west,
embrace our
cunning trap.
kiss us with
your chicken pox,
psora for the clap.

Sailing back
from conquered lands
bearing gifts of gold.
rape and carnage
darkened sun
the story won't be told.

- Acute stitches in the left side of the head, at the junction of the parietal and temporal bones.
- Dull sticking pain in the left side on the occiput.
- Pulsating throbbing externally on the head, with stitches in the temples.
- Some stitches in the right malar bone.
- Stitches as from knives in the right cheek.
- Drawing pain in the left side of the lower jaw, ending in a stitch.
- Constant violent stitches in the throat.
- Stitches in the left hypochondriac region.
- Stitches in the neck of the bladder, after urinating.
- Cutting, while urinating, as though something biting passed from.
- Pain in the chest, stitches in the left side beneath the true ribs.
- Constant frequent stitches on the left side of the nape of the neck.
- Constant stitches, which at last become a continuous stitch, just beneath the right scapula.
- Sharp stitch on the top of the right shoulder, frequently returning.
- Violent painful stitches in the right upper arm.
- Frequent drawing-tearing stitches, extending from the left elbow to the wrist.
- Some violent stitches in the right thumb.
- Some stitches in the left thigh above the knee.
- Drawing pain in the knee, which ends in a stitch.
- Drawing stitches in the right leg, extending from the ankle up to the middle of the tibia.
- Violent jerking stitches in the outer side of the calf.
- Sharp stitches in the right ankle.
- Pain, ending in a sharp stitch, in a small spot on the back of the right foot.
- Itching stitches like fleabites in the skin of the thigh.
- Single sharp stitches in the right ankle joint.

The Point

- Dreams as if she would be stabbed with knives.
- Dreams: knives, keeping them ready for use
- Cutting in the bowels.
- Cutting when urinating as if something biting passed.
- Needle-like stitches in the nates, as though she sat upon needles.
- Sitting: on needles in rectum.
- Pricking: back, pins were.

Wooden ships on the water
pulleys turn
rotating.
oily wood that will not rot
hinges creak
joints aching.

Black knight syphilis stowaway,
hiding deep in hull.
Grinning, leering,
salivating,
waiting for the
cull.

Too late…
doorknob quietly turns
knight slinking through the door,
hugs a sailor
back from travels,
mates his woman
on the shore.

Venereal contract
love for money
pain and pleasure moan,
treponema
on her travels
wart to bubo,
brain to
bone.

French disease?
or English? Russian?
who can tell for sure.
obscure the point
of origin
hide guilt for
evermore.

Stuck to a Spot

- In the morning when standing absence of thought; he remains standing at one spot, and stares right in front of him without thinking.
- While he lay asleep on his back, he dreamt that some one was lying on him; from anxiety he could not fetch his breath nor cry out.
- Laziness for work.
- Laziness and dislike to movement.
- The symptoms almost all appear while sitting.
- Rheumatic stiffness of the whole left side of the back, from the nape of the neck down to the sacrum, with intolerable pain on the slightest motion, not noticed during rest.
- Contractions between scapulae: causing immobility.
- Pain in the abdomen, a griping in the left side of the umbilicus, in a small spot.

Hardness

- Hardened mucus in the canthi of the right eye.
- A hardened pimple with a white tip in the right eyebrow, with very sore pain when touched.
- Tonsillitis with rheumatism.
- Desire for apples.

Narrow Minded

- Delusion: everything seems too narrow
- Morose mood; he speaks little.
- Rigidity.
- Contemptuousness.
- Strong desire to criticize and to despise everything.
- Indolent, obstinate, fretful.
- Intellectual.
- Vivid dreams of scientific subjects.
- Weakness of memory.
- Weakness of memory; he forgets what he has just read, and no longer remembers familiar names.
- Sensation as if the brain were loose and moved on every step.

Expansion

- Sensation of swelling and protrusion of the eyes, the lids seem too short to cover them; therewith a sensation of loss of sleep, with yawning and stretching the whole day.
- Yawning and stretching, with comfortable sensation.
- Stretching of the upper limbs, with yawning.

Prickling pains.
stitching pains.
grinding to a halt.
darting
stitching needles,
ending in a point.
gnawing pains.
drawing pains.
fibres are too
short.

Rigid joints
now cease turning
agonising warmth.
fingers gnarl
into a hook,
thighs contract,
deformed.

Rheumatics scream,
tonsils howl,
spongy bones complain.
abcess gnaws
at soft palates,
suppurating
brain.

Growing pains
stretch a limb,
yawn constricts a mind.
bulging eyes
contract their lids,
soul caught in a
bind.

- Growing pains.
- Pain, like growing-pains, in the right thigh.
- Dilated pupils.
- The face is swollen, red, and painful, for several days.

Tearing Apart (at the joint)

- Dreams of fights.
- Tearing stitch in the right side of the head going towards the frontal bone.
- A drawing tearing in the forepart of the forehead.
- Tearing in the right side of the occiput.
- Tearing in the whole of the left side of the head.
- Tearing from the left side of the head at the frontal bone downwards into the cheek muscles.
- Tearing in the outer margin of the left concha.
- Tearing in the left ear.
- Tearing in the outer border of the left ear cartilage.
- Tearing in the upper molar teeth of the left side.
- Drawing and tearing posteriorly under the axilla down the right side of the spine to the last true rib.
- Tearing stitches on the posterior border of the right scapula.
- Painful drawing tearing in the left upper and forearm into all the fingers, but particularly continued and permanent in the left wrist joint.
- Frequent drawing tearing stitches from the left elbow into the wrist joint.
- Tearing in the right forearm extending into the wrist-joint.
- Pressive like tearing in the left wrist joint.
- Drawing tearing from the middle of the left thigh to the knee.
- Twitching tearing in the right thigh from its middle to the knee.
- Tearing obtuse stitches from the middle of the left tibia to the toes.
- Drawing tearing stitches from the middle of the right tibia to the knee.
- Tearing long-drawn stitches in the right leg, extending from the dorsum of the foot to the knee.
- Betwixt the tibia and fibula shooting tearings to the patella, so violent as to jerk the leg upwards.
- Long drawing, tearing stitches from the right tarsus into the knee.

Relevant Rubrics (Complete Repertory)

- Mind; anxiety; constriction of; stomach, in
- Mind; audacity

Muscles shrink,
synovials shrivel,
tendons cringe in pain.
hardened nodes
exostosed brain,
criticise
constrain.

Narrow view and
narrow mind,
attitudes congealing.
disagreements,
disobedience,
now a riot's
brewing.

Burning streets
foul secretions,
rooted to the spot.
abscess bursts
truncheon strikes,
now we have to
stop.

Black knight syphilis rages on
will science save the day?
analysing,
knife dissecting,
hard facts only
just one way.

Lay back Eve,
crunch your apple
hard and round and small.
snakey syphilis
winds its way
into a compact ball.

- Mind; censorious, critical
- Mind; contemptuous
- Mind; contrary
- Mind; defiant
- Mind; delirium; look fixed on one point
- Mind; delusions, imaginations; narrow, everything is too
- Mind; discontented, displeased, dissatisfied
- Mind; disobedience
- Mind; dreams; battles
- Mind; dreams; cutting
- Mind; dreams; cutting; knife, of being cut with a
- Mind; dreams; fights
- Mind; dreams; frightful
- Mind; dreams; intellectual
- Mind; dreams; knives
- Mind; dreams; knives; pierced with
- Mind; dreams; luck, of bad
- Mind; dreams; misfortune, of
- Mind; dreams; murder
- Mind; dreams; murdered, of being
- Mind; dreams; nightmare
- Mind; dreams; quarrels, strife
- Mind; dreams; riots
- Mind; dreams; scientific
- Mind; dreams; stabbed
- Mind; fear; general; exertion, of
- Mind; haughty
- Mind; malicious, vindictive
- Mind; meditation; general
- Mind; misanthropy
- Mind; mocking; general
- Mind; morose, sulky, cross, fretful, ill-humor, peevish
- Mind; obstinate, headstrong
- Mind; sit; inclination to
- Mind; slander, disposition to
- Mind; staring, thoughtless
- Mind; thoughts; vanishing, loss of; standing, while
- Mind; wearisome

Sacred wood
as sacred should,
cure our dark afflictions.
from fight and tight
to love and light,
relaxing our
constrictions.

Sister Thuja
tree of life,
growing wide and tall,
I'm not like you,
sprouting warts,
I'm tough
condensed
and
small.

Sycosis grows
on wings of wood,
soul floating to the sky.
the secret of
proliferation;
duplicate
to multiply.

I sold my soul
wood for metal,
changed my mode of life.
to fabricate
or emulate
a pulley, hinge
or knife.

- Generalities; constricted sensation; internal
- Generalities; constricted sensation; external
- Generalities; contractions, strictures, stenoses; general
- Generalities; exostoses
- Generalities; food and drinks; apples; amel
- Generalities; food and drinks; apples; desires
- Generalities; growth; length, in, too fast
- Generalities; motion; agg.

You reach for skies
I grasp for roots,
one we cannot be.
syphilis and sycosis
night and day
in rivalry.

From sun so bright
to deadly night
shade
of metal,
cold.
Sacred wood.
Ironwood.
Can thou heal my soul?

From Fracastoro's 'Syphilis'

The curse

"Then they lay out their hard tack and jars of their country's wine on a grassy bank: next they investigated whether any humans were living there: some gazed in wonder at the river's deep yellow stream and sifted the gold-mingled sand. It so happened that large flocks of birds were all the time flying through the shady branches of the trees, ornate birds, their blue flashing wings contrasting with their red beaks, who passed untroubled through their native grove's wilderness. When the bands of young men saw these flying among the lofty trees they snatched up their hollow bronze pieces which shudder with terrifying booms and the missiles which imitate the flame-bearing thunderbolt, your invention, Vulcan, when you armed the Teutons, when you brought Jove's weapons to mortals. And there's no delay, each marks out for himself a particular bird, they kindle the enclosed material, charcoal from willow, sulphur and saltpetre, with a spark preserved in tow. The tinder catches light, the fiery force, hemmed in, suddenly pours out raging and as it quickly bursts through the barrier, simultaneously it drives out the bullet thrust inside. This flies through the air whistling; and winged creatures lay everywhere through the glades, knocked down, lifeless: the air flickered with fire accompanied by great thunderings which caused all the forest, the winding shore and the sea from its deepest depths to reverberate and echo. Some of the birds retreated, flocking together in terror, into the dense grove and to the high rocks. From their highest point one (marvellous to say) sang a dreadful prophecy and filled the men's ears with terrifying words, speaking like this.

"You who have done violence to the birds of the Sun, his sacred flying creatures, you men of Hesperia, hear now what almighty Apollo prophesies, what he declares to you by our mouth... and after battling against men on all sides, many of you bury dead bodies in a foreign land. Ships will be lost so that few of you will make for your home lands; others retraversing the mighty seas will search for comrades in vain. Nor will Cyclopes be wanting in this hemisphere. Discord herself will drag your crews into mad and murderous disputes; and a day lies in wait for you, close at hand, when, your bodies filthy with an unknown disease, you will in your wretchedness demand help of this forest until you repent of your crimes." She spake no more and with a dreadful hiss hid in the dense shadows. A shiver suddenly ran through their bones, and every man grew pale and their blood fled in chill terror. Then they prayed in earnest to the sacred birds and the Gods; first with vows and supplication they revered the Sun and the rural deities, who kept the sacred grove: they prayed for peace, and again they paid respect to Ophyre and the river.

...It so happened that a feast day occurred in the locality and they were preparing to perform annual rites to Sun the Avenger in a shady grove. The whole band, Spaniards and people of Ophyre, had assembled. Here in a hollow valley, on the grassy green of a bank, a great number of folk stood, set apart, mothers and their menfolk milling together, the masses and the aristocracy, boys and old men, all with melancholy hearts and hideous bodies, scaly with scabs, flowing with pus. As they milled around, a priest in white robes cleansed them with purifying waters and with a branch of leafy Guaiacum.

The cure

...I must now sing of the Gods' great gifts and of the sacred tree brought from an unknown world, which alone has moderated, relieved and ended suffering.

...Happy the poet to whom God has granted so much. But for me it is enough to recall the powers of a single tree and its use: in what manner it was discovered and how over that vast expanse of sea it arrived a stranger to live in our air.

...the land is fertile in gold, but made far richer by one tree - they call this in the sounds of their native speech Guaiacum. The tree itself is smooth and being huge spreads from its high top a huge canopy ever green, tresses of arbute leaves ever in place. Its nut, which is small but bitter, hangs down from the branches and clings to the leaves in great quantities. The tree's timber is difficult to master, the wood is almost like hard iron; when burnt it exudes a sticky resin. The colour of a dissected piece is complex. On the outside bark it is smooth and green like laurel; the next layer is pale like box; but the middle is dark brown with a hint of black, a cross between walnut and ebony. If it were red next then it could equal the rainbow with its varied colours. That foreign race adores this tree and is very eager in its efforts to rear it: with this the hills and open plains far and wide, with this every field is clothed: nor is anything more sacred to them or of more important use; for all hope lies in it against this plague which the heavens have there made eternal. Casting away the bark they beat the strong branches with great force or they file them into minute particles and they lay these in the fountains pure water, until the moisture has been absorbed by the powdered wood for a day and a night while steeping. Then they cook it...

... For with this froth they anoint any abscess there is anywhere on the body, any sore which is eating away the diseased frame.

...immediately that sacred draught, like ambrosia, restores and nurses your strength and the fasting limbs allow it to carry nourishment into the secret places.

...At the same time the plague vanishes into the vacant air, and astonishing to say blisters no longer appear; and now all the ulcers are gone, now the pain has gone, leaving the limbs strong, and youth in its first flower returns; and now the new moon comes back having travelled its circuit.

Coming home

With these and other stories, covering many topics, the peoples who had mingled together from opposite parts of the globe away the time. Meanwhile the ships which had been sent back to Europe's loved shores, when they had retracked across the wide seas, brought astonishing news: widely (oh the hidden fates of the Gods) this same contagion was spreading in the sky of Europe, and harassing cities dismayed by lack of remedies. Indeed a more serious rumour ran though all the ships that the fleet, and no scant number of its youth, were in the grip of this same illness, all their limbs wasting away. So not forgetting that the birds of ill omen had sung that a time would come when help would be requested from the wood, straightway after praying to the nymphs and the Sun to be sympathetic they prepared to collect branches from the virgin forest and pieces of trunk from the lofty grove and took up cups of the medicine according to the native rite; by this favour they finally repelled the savage contagion. Moreover not forgetting their homeland they ordered the Gods' gifts and this blessed tree to be brought to our shores, in the hope perhaps of repelling the kindred disease from this clime: even the fates offered Westerlies to speed them on their way and Apollo breathed on them easing their path. You were the first, Spaniards, to receive the favours of the Gods, marvelling at the help on hand. Now Guaiacum is known to French and Germans and Slavs, it rejoices in the world of Italy, it has now already been carried into every part of Europe. Hail great tree sown from a sacred seed by the hand of the Gods, with beautiful tresses, esteemed for your new virtues: hope of mankind, pride and new glory from a foreign world; most happy tree, if only the holy powers had wished you to have been born under our heaven and to grow amid this race of men belonging to the Gods, sacred with everlasting wood. Yet you yourself shall be known even in these parts and you will also be sung under our heavens, wherever through our song the muses can make you travel by the lips of men."

Guaiacum Synthesis

Verb

Sensation:
Contracting to a point - stitching.

Function:
Expansion and stretching - tearing.

Sensation and function:
Contracting and expanding. Stitching and tearing.

Image

Narrow mind. Dissecting rigid intellect.
Contracted personality.
Fights, riots and revolution. Tearing apart rigid contracted structures.

Hepar Sulphuris Calcareum

Hepar Sulphuris Calcareum

"...After you have seen a great many cases you will find that you have killed some of them. If our medicines were not powerful enough to kill folks, they would not be powerful enough to cure sick folks. It is well for you to realize that you are dealing with razors when dealing with high potencies. I would rather be in a room with a dozen Negroes slashing with razors than in the hands of an ignorant prescriber of high potencies. They are means of tremendous harm, as well as of tremendous good."
(Kent, *Lectures on Materia Medica; 'Hepar Sulphur'*)

This well-known and cutting quote from Kent has caused some contention. Sensibilities are offended. Some regard it as an abusive racist comment, while others balk at the possibility that a positive medicine is capable of such intense violence. This paragraph also reflects the controversy between opposing camps of homœopaths regarding the issue of potency.

Was Kent a genius or a politically incorrect bigot? Was he a combination of both? Or was he simply prone to fiery outbursts?

Let us examine the context.

Hepar means **combination**, and the remedy Hepar sulphuris calcareum is a chemical combination of calcium carbonate and sulphur. It has some of the properties of both, but is very different from either. It was known before Hahnemann's time as "Liver of Sulphur" and used as an external remedy for itch. Hahnemann proposed Hepar as a remedy for mercury poisoning. His unique preparation of Hepar is described in *The Chronic Diseases:*

"A mixture of equal parts of finely powdered, clean oyster shells and quite pure flowers of sulphur is kept for ten minutes at a white heat in a hermetically closed crucible and afterwards stored up in a well-corked bottle."

Hepar is prepared in a crucible, a closed furnace. In go the smouldering yellow flowers of sulphur; in goes the cool calcareous oyster shell. Seal the oven, light the gas, raise the temperature to 'high'. Then sit back and wait for alchemy to combust.

At this point we may meditate on Hahnemann's reasons for choosing such an unusual

concoction. It seems that this alchemical process mimics a natural occurrence. Volcanic sulphur and lime, locked together many miles under the surface of the earth, are subjected to extreme **pressure** and intense **heat**. Like a raging abscess, boiling lava seeks a **vent**.
These two substances, sulphur and calcarea, are in many ways polar opposites.
They represent contrasts of heat and cold, fire and air, day and night, conscious and subconscious. Hahnemann has taken two **opposing** energies and forced them together. What can we expect from this alchemical brew?

To **penetrate** into the inner nature of this remedy we will begin our study with the generals. Once the pattern becomes clear we can **probe** the mentals searching for a deeper understanding.

The Hepar patient is both **chilly** and aggravated by cold. The **chilliness** is **intense**, not the normal lack of vital heat common to many remedies. He wants to be **wrapped** in warm clothing and may wear thermal underwear and a winter coat in the summer.
He wants the **heating turned up** fully and the **windows closed**. Others may find this oppressive heat difficult to bear. In contrast, Hepar has also been noted to kick the covers off in winter.

To avoid the **intrusion** of cold air Hepar must **keep covered**. Blankets are drawn tightly around the **neck**. It is characteristic of Hepar that a finger or toe **probing** out of the covers causes immediate aggravation and must be hurriedly withdrawn behind **protective** layers. Naturally they will continue to repeat this process of **sticking** the finger out and in. Pathology tends to itch its own scratch.

If we conjure up this image of the sick Hepar – windows closed, room overheated, covers drawn closely around - we are reminded of the original preparation of this remedy.
Shut in a sizzling crucible, sulphur and calcarea are totally **insulated** from the cooling environment. The furnace is **sealed** and the heat is on.

Hepar's most aggravating modality is the **cold dry wind**, which **pierces** right through him. Wind is air in motion, driven by differentials of temperature, oppositions of heat and cold. Wind moves, stirs and **penetrates**. It portrays the dramatic tension between the elements of fire and air. The nature of dry cold wind is **sharper** and more **cutting** than other winds. In Chinese medicine it is associated with **sudden** and **intense** conditions.

In opposition to this cold (Air) element, the eruptions of Hepar possess the characteristics of fire. Blistering boils, bubbling abscesses and sizzling pustules burst to the surface like erupting volcanoes.

The Hepar tension between heat and cold is further represented by food desires. On one hand they crave **spicy food**, **mustard** and **whisky**, and on the other they desire sour food and vinegar (sour relates to oxygen, cold and sharp).

Hepar and Fat

Hepar is one of the main remedies desiring fat. To understand our remedies it is useful to study their physiology in a wider context. Insulation is provided by the fatty adipose layer under the skin. Fat provides protection, especially from the cold.

Fat has two major roles in the body - storage and insulation. These functions belong to the Earth element. Earth (bricks and mortar) is used to build and insulate our houses. Hepar experiences problems with the functions of insulation and storage (emaciation).

Fat represents congealed energy. We may think of energy as physiological currency. Glucose in the blood relates to cash in the pocket, always at hand and ready to use. Glycogen in the liver is money in the bank, safely stored for a time of need, but more difficult to get hold of. We use insulin like a credit card, to release energy and money. Fat is similar to a house, providing insulation, investment and long term storage, but cumbersome and difficult to liquidate. Hepar, like Sulphur, has problems associated with fat. Like Calc carb, it lacks the protective shell of home. The combination represents fat as an insulating shell.

The Hepar patient is generally characterised by a great **sensitivity**. In the repertory we find oversensitivity to all external stimuli, including mental and emotional impressions. This oversensitive disposition indicates that the Hepar patient is lacking **protection**. They have no barriers to the external world. They wrap themselves with clothes and blankets to compensate for the **insulation** that they are missing internally. Their nerves are described as raw and bare, **exposed** to the environment. Ulcers penetrate **protective** layers of skin and **fat**.

The pains of Hepar are severe and very **sharp**. Eruptions, boils or abscesses are full of sharp pains. Deep ulcers erode protective layers, exposing painfully raw nerves. Ulcer pains are described as sharp and **piercing**, like **jagging** sticks. The suffering is intense. These pains depict the theme of **penetration**.

We can now define the sensation and function of Hepar. The main sensation and function are '**exposed and penetrated, must insulate**', and the reciprocal '**insulated, must penetrate**'. This pattern is best illustrated by the patient repeatedly poking a finger or toe out of the covers and then hastily retreating. The need to penetrate may take various forms. They may stick things in their nose or ears, fantasise about rape, or possess knives. The need to insulate is illustrated by Hepar's affinity to encysted tubercles in the lungs. These tubercles are covered with a calcium wall, thus protecting the rest of the body.

Sensation and function can reverse themselves, as they represent a continuous cycle of opposites. Where Hepar perceives insulation it will try to penetrate. Where Hepar senses exposure, it will over-insulate. This cycle plays itself out on all levels; physical, mental and emotional. One example is Hepar's capacity to remove foreign projectiles. This is in accord with its function of 'must **insert**'. The sensation of jagged sticks materialises as injuries from **needle** tips, **bullets** and **splinters**. Once the need to be penetrated and **enclosed** is cured by potentised Hepar, the external projectile is no longer necessary.
A vent is found and the intruder is expelled.

The lack of insulation is also reflected in Hepar's emotional makeup. All external stimuli are intensely amplified by the overexposed sensibilities. Hepar is sensitive to people, sad stories, cruelty and noise. A typical Hepar response to this oversensitivity may be emotional insulation, an attempt to 'cover up'. Another response may be intense irritability, anger and abuse. The anger may be fiery and explosive, but the abuse is cold and cutting.

The aggressive behaviour of Hepar may be very **impulsive**. The physiological equivalent of impulse is reflex action, where there is no time, or ability, for a message to travel up the spine for the mind to consider. Impulse means action without thought. We are all subject to irrational impetuosity. However, our intellect, a restricting influence, forbids rash transgressions. Like a bursting abscess, impulsive Hepar emotions penetrate inhibitory intellectual insulation.

This relationship between erupting emotions and protective intellect parallels the relationship between body and mind. The junction of these forces, emotion and intellect, is represented by the neck. It is therefore significant that Hepar has a great affinity with the neck and throat. They feel as if they had swallowed a **fish bone** or **splinter** causing **stitching** pains in the throat. Hepar often pulls the covers tightly around the neck, or grasps the throat while coughing. It is apparent that the **throat** and **neck** are focal points of Hepar. Body tightly covered, head probing outwards, this narrow connection between head and body represents the weak link of this remedy.

This head - body conflict is portrayed by Hepar's components, sulphur and calcarea. Sulphur represents the intellectual or conscious aspect - a theoriser disgusted by his physical body and base emotions. Calcarea's weak mind is unable to restrain emotions, fears and anxieties, which surface from a dark subconscious. Hepar is the explosive combination of Calcarea's free floating emotions with Sulphur's tendency to override feelings with intellect.

One of the strangest impulses of Hepar is the impulse to kill. A sudden urge compels him to kill his best friend. Desire to kill is unusual, but an urge to kill one's **best friend** is rare. These urges are unthinkable to most people.

Hepar's desire to kill is often by **stabbing.** Colonel Hepar in the oven with a **knife**. Kent says: "A barber has an impulse to cut the throat of his patron while in the chair". Immediately a whole genre of spaghetti westerns spring to mind. Red and white spiral on the door-post, barbaric barber finely sharpening his razor on a leather strap, eyeing the exposed neck of his customer. The sticking fish bone has become a slashing knife, threatening to sever head from body.

Hepar may also set fire to people or things. Even stranger is the impulse of the Hepar mother to throw her baby into the fire. Rather than **hug** the baby, she wants to **burn** him, or in other cases set **fire** to herself. This is a dreadful thought to contemplate. Closer than the attachment to a best friend, the mother child **bond** is the closest **connection** of all. More then any other, this symptom symbolises the intense turmoil within.

Under what circumstances would a mother burn her own child? Why would a person kill his best friend? Under normal circumstances, such phenomena are rare. In the absence of internal pathology, these acts could only be responses to **threats** of extreme violence or abuse. Predicaments such as war, torture and concentration camps come to mind; situations of extreme **danger** where there is **no escape** or **outlet**. In the case of morbid pathology, these hazardous situations exist only in the mind. Mimicking the **subterraneous conditions** of **extreme heat and pressure**, Hepar creates its own **hell**.

Imagine the following scenario. Young Mr Sulphur meets pretty Miss Calcarea, courting her with warm affections, a bottle of wine, yellow flowers. They follow each other around and seem to get on well. A rosy future awaits the couple, a warm and secure **union** as the Calc-sulph family. Little more then compliments and mutual appreciation will be needed to kindle the flames of love. Any minor irritations are discussed, discharged and ventilated. Yet the same couple living in the ghetto compose a very different story. Poverty, violence and misery prevail. Life is tough. The marriage of Calc and Sulph is rushed, forced forward by an early pregnancy. Another child follows, then five more. Work is scarce, money scarcer. Home is a one room windowless flat, boiling in summer and freezing in winter.

The loan sharks arrive, followed by police and organised crime. The heat is on, pressure too intense to bear. There is no way out. A situation like this must find a vent. Arguments escalate to violence, and alcohol blows the tension. Lovers have mutated to enemies through adverse circumstance.

It is important to realise that this violent turmoil may **erupt** in situations that seem superficially healthy. Like a deceptively wholesome tooth filled with explosive pus, the anger of Hepar can be deeply suppressed. On the surface they may project a shiny enamel **positiveness**, like an ill-matched 'happy couple' who have not spoken for years. But underneath a raging abscess of hatred is on the boil, fuelling long-term abuse and cruelty. Such anger often **bursts out** during bouts of drinking, an impulsive angry knife severing an **apparently close family**.

I now refer back to Kent's controversial comment from the beginning of this chapter:

"..It is well for you to realise that you are dealing with razors when dealing with high potencies. I would rather be in a room with a dozen Negroes slashing with razors than in the hands of an ignorant prescriber of high potencies. They are means of tremendous harm, as well as of tremendous good."

This comment may not be politically correct, but I do not believe that Kent intended to discredit any race. This situation was not uncommon in 19th century Chicago. Whatever our opinion, it was Kent's genius to include this highly descriptive image of Hepar in his lecture. Enclosed and surrounded, **threatened** with sharp knives, **no way out.**

Hepar the Peacemaker

True to its name, Hepar joins or separates non-unified bonds. F.E. Gladwin, in her book "*People of the Materia Medica*" relates the story of three 'friends' in "Hepar the Peacemaker". Silica and Mercury are inimical, and don't get along very well. This inimical relationship often exists between two remedies that are externally similar but internally very different. Silica, the timid intellectual, and Mercury, the impulsive repulsive, are forced to co-exist in the materia medica due to superficial similarities. Hepar acts as an intercurrent and resolves the differences between these antagonistic remedies. When these two opposing entities are forcibly united, Hepar sulphuris calcareum provides a third intermediary.

Hepar is a remedy for all three miasms. Sulphur and Calcarea are naturally psoric. It is the non union of these contrary forces that creates affinity to the syphilitic and sycotic miasms.

Interestingly, a few of the Hepar cases I have seen had three marriages. One described her first husband as Mr. Fire, and the second as Mr. Ice.

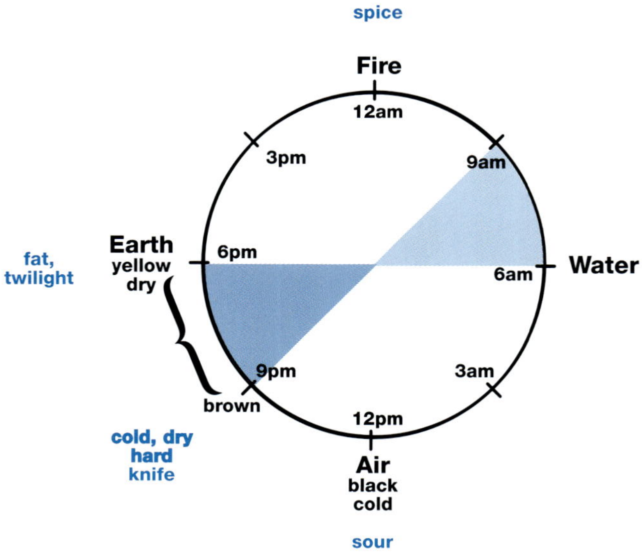

Hepar Sulph Synthesis

Verb

Sensation:
Exposed.

Function:
Must insulate.

Sensation:
Insulated, sealed;
Function:
Must penetrate – insert.

Form:
Two opposing entities forcefully conjoined. Hepar – to join.

Noun

Knife. Fish bone. Needle. Splinter.

Image

Fire and air – wind.
Contradictory forces with no outlet.
Sealed volcano.
Insulated eruption seeking a vent.
Surrounded by razors. No way out.
Head contradicting body, mind contradicts emotion – cut throat.
Positive exterior – peacemaker.

Mercurius

Working with Mercury

From Allen's *Encyclopedia*

"He was emaciated and cachectic, and looked prematurely old.
Great emaciation. Body wasted. Cachectic condition".

"It is certain that the children of the workers are affected with the mercurial poisoning; although it may be from the poison carried by the clothing. One child of a woman-worker was badly nourished, and when a year old had no teeth. The children of the workers were pale, cachectic, and scrofulous; while in the same locality, the children of those who did not work at silvering mirrors were usually healthy. The children of the workers are very commonly affected by scrofula rachitis, and tuberculosis".

"A daughter, born during her mercurialism, was very small, only learned to walk when three years old, and never grew to be more than four feet in height; there was kyphoscoliotic curvature of the spine, the head was drawn to the chest and somewhat to the left side; there was very imperfect development of the muscle and bone".

"This worker had four children by his first wife, who was also employed in the factory; all were sickly; one son died of gangrene of both feet; the three other children and the wife died of consumption; the second wife and her children also died of consumption; the children of the third wife were healthy except the one born after she was employed in the works; all three wives died in consumption".

"A child of one of the workers, a year old, had trembling of the arms, moderate stomatitis, and ptyalism; the child was pale, but well nourished, even fat, and intelligent".

"Fatal consumption. One woman, who had been healthy and had three healthy children, died of tuberculosis".

"Among five hundred patients suffering from caries, necrosis or exostosis of the bones, there is no case known of it occurring among the workers in Mercury".

"Syphilis is extremely rare among the workers in Mercury, especially remarkable since the sexual desire is usually excited; several physicians who practiced in Furth, where the factories are, and who had a large practice among syphilitics, could not remember a single case of syphilis among the workers".

"Within thirty years, more than hundred persons in Erlangen and four or five times as many in Furth, have been treated for constitutional mercurial poison; and though these cases have increased sexual desire in consequence of Mercury and, without doubt are not particular about their associations, since among them the belief is universal that Mercury protects them from syphilis, no case has been known to occur".

"The first symptom was persistent diarrhoea, which lasted profusely eight days, and ceased after she stopped work; after a year and a half there appeared tremors with loss of appetite and diarrhoea, followed by falling out of the hair; on stopping work and using baths the tremors disappeared in four weeks, and the hair grew again; after returning to work the teeth began to be gray, though she daily scoured them with charcoal; afterwards she was attacked with weakness, vertigo, uneasy sleep with heavy dreams, loss of memory, affections of the mouth, which she treated with alum, and increased decay of the teeth; after a time the tremors reappeared and gradually becomes worse, as also did the headache and sleepiness; afterwards she had palpitation of the heart and hiccough, at times so violent that she had to be held by several people; after leaving the work she became better, but the tremors did not entirely leave her, and were especially aggravated by any vexation or other emotional excitement; the gums were somewhat atrophied and retracted from the teeth; teeth of a grayish-brown color; copper color of the roof of the palate and uvula; slight tremors of the extremities and of the tongue, especially noticeable in speech; the right posterior cervical gland swollen; rheumatic pains in both upper arms; profuse perspiration at night and easily becoming chilly; the patient had had two children, the first four weeks too early; the child was weak, and died when a year and a half old".

Mercurius Analysis

Can't Find Place – Must Move

- Towards evening, an uneasiness that did not permit him to remain in any place; he could not remain sitting two minutes; he was forced to change; also he was unable to remain lying on account of the jerking in the limbs; also at night he kept constantly rising; with jerking of the head and throwing about of the arms during sleep.
- No rest in any place, constantly anxious.
- Extreme restlessness all night, at one time he stood up because he had no rest while lying, then he lay down because walking was intolerable, and so he had no rest.
- An almost irresistible desire to take a distant journey.
- Almost uncontrollable desire to travel far away.
- Homesickness, or desire to travel; wants to go abroad.
- Desire to flee, with nightly anxiety and apprehension.
- Delusions, imaginations: home: away from, is
- Mind; wander; desires to
- Speech & voice; speech; wandering
- A frightful dream, in which he started up and thought he was not in his own house, sat up in bed and talked about a far-distant village.
- He does not know where he is.
- Forgot the names of persons and places, and was frequently at a loss in endeavoring to recollect the persons to whom he had lent his tools.
- Chaotic.
- Confusion of mind: loses his way in well-known streets
- Recognize: does not: house, his own
- Recognize: does not: relatives, his
- Worse from the warmth of the bed so that he is forced to uncover; but after he uncovers and cools off he gets worse again, so that he has difficulty in keeping comfortable.
- General tremors.
- Involuntary tremors.
- Mercurial tremors affect the muscles which are usually under the control of the will, so that one is never master of his own motions. On attempting to respond the muscles begin to tremble and twitch excessively; they frequently make all sorts of motions, as in chorea, before the desired motion is affected, or are sometimes affected with violent convulsive motions, which also involve neighboring groups of muscles.

Mercury Shatter Me

Where from mercury, where to?

A single globule of liquid metal rolls across the table, fugitive from a broken thermometer. Hydrargyrum, silver
water, makes its bid for freedom. One hundred degrees from boil to freeze was all the space it had. Gaining speed it reaches the edge, sharp breath before a final leap. Even as it falls the defiant droplet holds its shape, bound by an enormous surface tension. Vivacious we run, united we fall. And then - splat! The globule explodes into a thousand tiny beads. Scattered, shattered, rolling, fleeing, it's every drop for itself. Mischievous particles propel themselves in every direction, impudent young beads lose track of their mothers, estranged sisters rush a frenzy. Repulsed relatives clash and quarrel, refusing to amalgamate. Galloping globules regard each other as enemies, to be clashed with, contradicted, fought against. The idea that this vivacious chaos was once merged in a sea of harmony is lost forever. Six billion scattered individuals enveloped by the tight metallic membrane of ego are all that is left of a shattered unity.

What now, mercury, what now?

Restless travellers wander abroad, attracted by the love of home. Flat ulcers spread in all directions, oozing greasy deposits from a rotting base. Compulsive hydrophobics wash their hands, putrid abscesses discharging filthy pus. Beggars slurp dirty mugs of tea, fatty globules floating to the surface. Disgusting degenerates leer repulsively, stooping to lick blood and spit from the road. Moaning livers store multiple toxicities, coagulated clots occluding corroded arteries. Hydrocephalic children gush watery saliva, seeping oily perspiration with no relief. Worms crawl and creep vaginas, pointless noses fail to lead the way. Rotten teeth invade puffy tongues, rolling stones abuse a mouth. Epileptics jerk and tremble, scalps tight against bony skulls. Jesting jokers pull a nose, retracted gums exposing long black teeth. Impudent children taunt maliciously, abused anorexics mutilate in self-contempt. Oily haired youth roam the streets, oozing odours of violence. Wives quarrel husbands, husbands abuse friends. Hackers surf the nightly net, communicating contradiction. Precocious egos cut their nose to spite your face, lost drivers search in vain for home. Tubercular travellers gorge greasy sandwiches, emaciated prostitutes scorn the night. Geniuses misplace memories, blank words, forget dates.

Water

The name: Mer-cury – sea
Hydrargyrum – silver water.

- Sees water running where there is none.
- Eyes water: objects were seen through, as if.
- Hydrophobia.
- Fear: water, of
- Dreams: water
- Dreams: water: danger from
- Dreams: water: falling into
- Dreams: water: flood, of a
- Rage, fury: water, sight of
- Considerable oedema of lower extremities.
- After suppression of foot sweat...uncontrollable desire to commit suicide.
- Mind; suicidal disposition; weeping, amel.
- So great was the violence of the trembling of his whole frame that he was nearly thrown out of a bath by it; much of the water was driven over the side of the tub.
- Worse in cold cloudy weather, or damp weather.
- Acute hydrocephalus.
- Left ear, a sensation as if cold water were running out.
- Morning sickness; profuse salivation, wets pillow in sleep.
- Mouth and tongue moist, and plenty of saliva, yet great thirst for cold water.
- The mouth was always full of water.
- Thirst for cold drinks, especially fresh water. Very great thirst for ice-cold water.
- Eructations: water, of: night
- Boiling: water, stools were
- Far more urine was passed than water had been drunk.
- Urine; watery, clear as water
- Water, prepuce were distended with
- Water: foot, as if: dipped into cold water: sole
- Chilliness, as if dashed with cold water.
- Vesicles full of water.

Confused accountants can't calculate alzheimers stare at unfamiliar children. Maniacal inmates strain straight jackets, frantic eyes rolling side to side. Merchants of deceit flash metallic smiles, flabby tongues wagging slander. Alcoholics reek revolting language from the bottom of their bottles, rambling revellers flaunting flashy knives. Restless anxiety paces the crossroads, thieves lurk the alleys, dreams lose their way. Dictatorial anarchists reproach rude rebels, impulsive misanthropics suppurate suicidal insanity. Wrecked tankers spew slick black lubricant on chaste blue seas, commerce smearing its sin. Chaos cradles death, death abuses life. Slimeball mercury hitches a ride on dentists and doctors, touching a gum, destroying a face, consuming a nose with cocaine.

And why?

Why, Mercury, why? Why seek to degrade the human race to its lowest possible salivating greasy gutter. Must you forever roam the earth like the scattered people of Babel? What lesson do you teach, what lesson must we learn? Is your purity too great to bear, untainted spotless silver innocence of wisdom? As Hahnemann purified mercury, so your spirit shines the pureness of life.

Until when, Mercury, until when? Dissolver of truth, winged messenger, alchemist of the double helix. Until when must you hide your shining countenance in greasy grime? Will you forever straddle the two faces, heat and cold, purified filth and oily water? Will the time come when you amalgamate virtue and profanity into the holy wholeness of life?
Amen.

Fat, Grease

- Obesity.
- Considerable emaciation.
- Excessive emaciation.
- Body wasted.
- Loss of their usual quantity of fatty matter, is very rapid.
- The albumin find in their places a certain fatty substance.
- The liver and kidneys are anaemic, enlarged, and show fatty degeneration.
- He has aversion to greasy food, butter.
- Food and drinks: fats and rich food: agg
- Food and drinks: fats and rich food: aversion
- Food and drinks: butter: aversion
- Food and drinks: bread and butter desires
- Food and drinks: butter: desires
- Craving for fat.
- Fat; hands
- Very profuse fatty and oily perspiration.
- Fatty kind of itch.
- Eruptions: scabies: fatty
- Hair: greasy
- Oily; skin.
- Nose; oily
- Face; greasy
- Hiccough as if he had swallowed boiling oil.
- Ulcers have a lardaceous base, looking as if spread over with a coating of lard.

Spread

- Spits a great deal and rubs it over the floor with her feet.
- Ulcers spread both in circumference and depth and secrete a yellow excoriating discharge.
- This tremor being altogether beyond the control of the patient and gradually spreading over the entire body.
- Food and drinks: bread and butter desires,
- Ulcers have a lardaceous base as if spread over with a coating of lard.
- The superficial ulceration is inclined to spread and become phagedenic; it is not deep but grows larger.
- Merc-c. is a great remedy for the superficial, eating, phagedenic ulcer.
- Lardaceous base in ulcers; flat ulcers, spreading ulcers.
- The ulcer spreads rapidly in extent, without penetrating into the flesh.

- But the most striking characteristic of the mercurial ulcer is its tendency to spread and the manner in which it enlarges itself; it generally spreads quickly, and there seems to be no limit to the size it may possibly attain.
- Eruptions: herpetic: spreading
- Vesicles on forepart and sides of glans penis; they eat deeply in and spread.
- Eczema on left hand gradually spreads to fingers and up to arm.
- Eruptive exanthema resembling roseola, which began first in the throat and face and from these parts spread all over the body.
- Mercurial sores...assume different forms as they spread.
- He was in the habit of crawling backwards and on his hands; he drank out of a dish, in order to bring the liquid more readily to his mouth.
- Radiating, spreading symptoms
- Face: shivering in and spreading from

Constrict

- She jumps up high both in the open air and in the house (like a wanton, unrestrained person)...so that the patient was obliged to be confined in a straitjacket.
- Bursting headaches, fullness of the brain, and constriction like a band.
- Constricted: brain were
- Band: head were constricted by a
- Great swelling redness in eyes, and constriction of the lids.
- Ears; contraction, constriction
- It is accompanied by violent constriction of the throat.
- Stomach feels constricted.
- Stomach; hard and tense; feels replete and constricted.
- Sensation of constriction in rectum.
- Constriction of chest.
- Constriction: prepuce
- Constriction: testes
- Constriction: vagina
- Constriction: external, sensation of
- Constriction: internal, sensation of
- Constriction: internal, sensation of: band, sensation of
- Constriction: internal, sensation of: bones
- Constriction: internal, sensation of: orifices, sphincter spasm
- Contractions, strictures, stenoses: inflammation, after

Offended, Offensive, Must Repel

- Repulsive mood.
- Odor of his mouth is so offensive and disgusting that it annoys everybody around him.
- Hatred: persons of, who had offended him
- He was very much offended if others laughed over a trifle.
- Frightful attacks of very irritable disposition. Very fretful and peevish.
- Morose and mistrustful all day; he treated his associates almost insultingly, and looked upon everybody as his worst enemy.
- Quarrels with everything; would above all have everything right.
- While taking a walk, he has a strong inclination to pinch the noses of the strangers he meets.
- Delirium; she uncovers herself at night, pulls the straw about, and scolds; during the day she jumps up high both in the open air and in the house (like a wanton, unrestrained person); she talks and scolds a great deal to herself, does not recognize her nearest relatives, spits a great deal and rubs it over the floor with her feet, then partly licks it up; she also frequently licks up cow dung and mud; she puts small stones into her mouth without swallowing them, and complains that they cut her intestines; she passes many clots of blood with the stool; she does violence to no one, but violently resists any one who attempts to touch her.
- He was foolish, played tricks, and made a fool of himself with senseless stuff; in the evening he made a fire in the stove (during the hot summer), laid swords across each other, placed lights in one corner of the room, boots in another, and all the time was fully in earnest.
- Was extremely averse to everything, even to music.
- Ailments from: disappointment, deception
- Ailments from: discords between: chief and subordinates
- Ailments from: discords between: relatives, friends
- Ailments from: egotism
- Anarchist: revolutionary
- Aversion: everything, to
- Aversion: family members, to
- Aversion: persons, to: certain
- Audacity
- Complaining: relations and surroundings, of
- Contradict, disposition to
- Contradiction: desires
- Contradiction: intolerant of
- Contrary
- Deceitful, sly: fraudulent

- Defiant
- Delusions, imaginations: enemy: everyone is an
- Delusions, imaginations: mutilated bodies, sees
- Delusions, imaginations: pursued, he is: enemies, by
- Dictatorial, domineering
- Disgust
- Dreams: disgusting
- Dreams: quarrels
- Dreams: revolution
- Dreams: riots
- Impolite
- Impulse, morbid
- Impulse, morbid: violence, to do
- Indiscretion
- Jesting: averse to
- Jesting: joke, cannot take a
- Kill, desire to: loved ones
- Kill, desire to: person that contradicts her
- Kill, desire to: sudden impulse to: husband, her beloved
- Reproaches others
- He is an offensive patient. We speak of mercurial odors. The breath especially is very fetid, and it can be detected on entering the room; it permeates the whole room. The perspiration is offensive; it has a strong, sweetish, penetrating odor. Offensiveness runs all through; offensive urine, stool and sweat; the odors from the nose and mouth are offensive. When Merc. is used in large doses and the patient is salivated he gives off these odors. One who has once smelt a salivated patient will remember the mercurial odor. I remember when I was a student, almost every room had the mercurial odor. Mercury was given till the gums were touched and salivation was produced. That odor is often an index to the use of Merc.
- Hemorrhage: blood: offensive
- Discharge: offensive: fetid
- Discharge: offensive: fetid: cheese, like
- Scurfy, syphilitic, pustular, moist, oozing, offensive eczema.

Enemy Of Self

- Seized with an almost uncontrollable desire to commit suicide.
- Anxiety driving her to suicide; thoughts of suicide; desire for death.
- Disgust of life. Much wretchedness and dejection of spirits.
- Is fearful that she may commit some wrong and kill herself.
- She puts small stones into her mouth without swallowing them, and complains that they cut her intestines.
- Great restlessness as if he had committed a great crime.
- He becomes disgustingly filthy and eats his own excrement.
- Disgusted with himself, has not courage to live.
- Disgust: himself, with
- Dreams: disgusting
- Anxiety: conscience, of
- Delusions, imaginations: crime: committed, he had
- Delusions, imaginations: criminal, that he is a
- Delusions, imaginations: fail, everything will
- Delusions, imaginations: hell: suffers the torments of, without being able to explain
- Delusions, imaginations: vagina, living things creep into, at night
- Discontented, displeased, dissatisfied: himself, with
- Dreams: swallowing pins

Surface Tension

Mercury has by far the highest surface tension of all liquids. Whereas the surface tension of water is 72.76 liquid dynes/cm, the surface tension of mercury is 487.00.

Surface tension, a condition existing at the free surface of a liquid, resembles the properties of an elastic skin under tension. The tension is the result of intermolecular forces exerting an unbalanced inward pull on the individual surface molecules; this is reflected in the considerable curvature at those edges where the liquid is in contact with the wall of a vessel.

The tendency of any liquid surface is to become as small as possible as a result of this tension, as in the case of mercury, which forms an almost round ball when a small quantity is placed on a horizontal surface.

When a drop rests on a flat surface, the surface tension between the liquid and the surface has an additional effect that causes a wetting fluid (such as water) to spread out, whereas a non-wetting fluid (such as mercury) will contract.

Mercurius Synthesis

Verb

Sensation:
Cannot find place (water).
Function:
Must wander.

Sensation:
Amalgamated. Contracted (water, purity).
Function:
Must repel; must scatter; must spread (fat, grime).

Form:

Triangle
Substance Nose, tibia, knife.

Image

Silver water – very high surface tension. Contracted to a droplet.
Fat spread thin on water. Pushing against a boundary.
Globules of fat scattered on water. Repulsion.
Purity repelling the 'oily grime of life'. Disgusting contradiction.

A Treatise of Mercury and the Philosophers Stone.

by Sir George Ripley, 1680

And now, my Son, that I may say something of the Philosophers Mercury, know that when thou hast put thy Water of Life to the Red man, who is our Magnesia, and to the White woman, whose name is Albifica, and they shall all have been gathered together into one, then you have the true Philosophers Mercury. For after that in this manner all is joyned with a Male and Female, then it is called the Philosophers Mercury, the Philosophers Water of Life…

…also Quicksilver, is Mercury; but I do not say, that common Quicksilver, is our Silver: as I said before, that Water of Life which is our Seed and first Matter, is our Mercury and our Spirit of Life, which is extracted out of the blessed land of Aethiopia, which is called Magnesia, and by many other names. Besides, my Son, know that there is no perfect generation, without corruption; for corruption causeth cleanliness, and cleanliness corruption.

…Son, ponder my words, otherwise if thou wanderest in the dark, that evil befalls thee from defect of light: See therefore that thou beest diligent in turning the Philosophick Wheel, that thou mayst make Water out of Earth, Air out of Water, Fire our of Air, and Earth out of Fire, and all this out of one Image and Root, that is, out of its own proper kind, and natural food wherewith its Life may be cherished without end. He who hath understanding, let him understand.

Glory to God Omnipotent.

FINIS.

From: 'The Mercury Language Reference Manual'

University of Melbourne, Australia, 1995 – 2002

Mercury is a new general-purpose programming language, designed and implemented by a small group of researchers at the University of Melbourne, Australia. Mercury is based on the paradigm of purely declarative programming, and was designed to be useful for the development of large and robust "real-world" applications.

Impurity declarations

...One important aim of Mercury's impurity system is to make the distinction between the pure and impure code very clear. This is done by requiring every impure predicate or function to be so declared, and by requiring every call to an impure predicate or function to be flagged as such. Predicates or functions that are implemented in terms of impure predicates or functions are assumed to be impure themselves unless they are explicitly promised to be pure.

Please note that the facilities described here are needed only very rarely. ...Any other use of 'impure' or 'semipure' probably indicates either a weakness in the Mercury standard library, or the programmer's lack of familiarity with the standard library. Newcomers to Mercury are hence encouraged to skip this section.

General Mercury

Mercury - metal of the sea, silver liquid, is held together by a surface tension much greater than that of water. This surface tension, combined with the power to amalgamate other metals into one alloy, characterises this liquid element with a powerful unifying quality. Yet mercury is vivacious by nature, animated activity that runs, rolls and frolics, slipping between grasping fingers or dancing the tune of temperature.

Next door resides its sombre neighbour Aurum, solidified sovereign sunshine in static state, and it's mother moon, Argentum. Planet Mercury circles the sun, orbiting a narrow comfort zone between scorching heat and a freezing solar system. The winged god of commerce and communication conveys solar messages to peripheral planets. In like manner, the astrological symbol of Mercury, lunar crest resting on a solar circle above the cross of matter, represents intuition communicating with knowledge via active intelligence.

Mercury favours the pituitary, which it can access by pulling a nose or consuming a palate. Located behind the centre brow, seat of navigation and intelligence, the pituitary nestles in the curve of the sella turcica, deriving its embryological roots from the hypothalamus above and the throat below. The binary solar rhythm of King pineal is transmitted to its glandular army by the mercurial General Pituitary.

Mercury and the Pituitary Gland

Pituitary glands taken post-mortem from Swedish dentists showed that the mercury level in the pituitary gland was, on average, 2.5 times (and in one case 169 times) that in the brain cortex.

Autopsies of former dental staff found levels of mercury in the pituitary gland averaged over 10 times that of controls.

The great majority of the body-burden of mercury – 87% – comes from dental amalgams, which continuously give off mercury vapor.

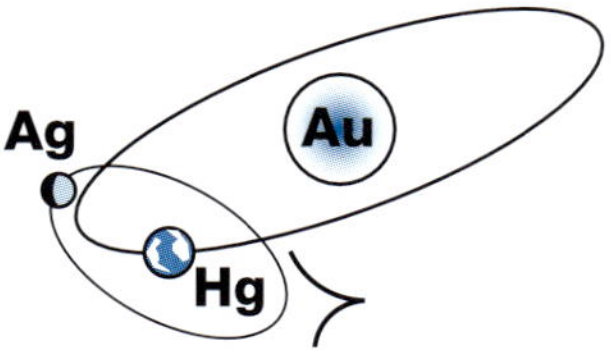

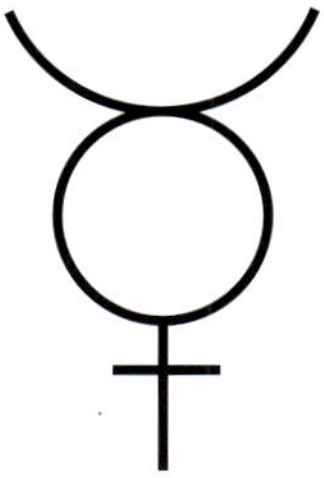

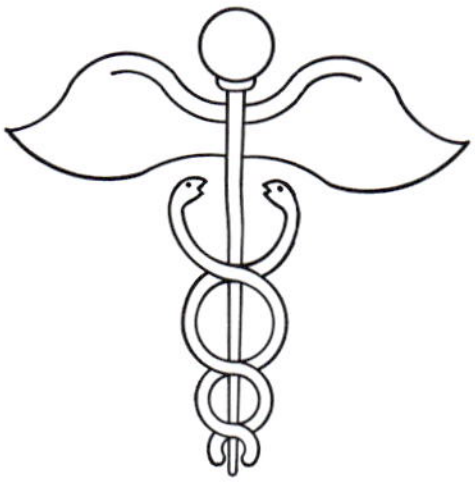

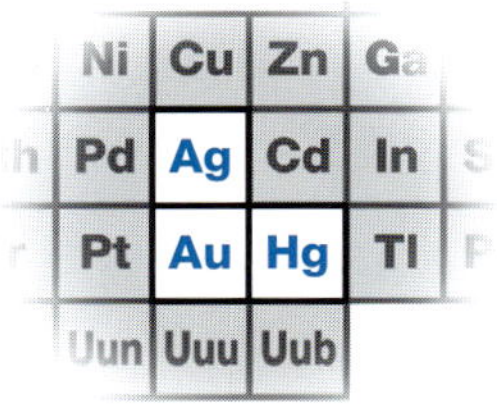

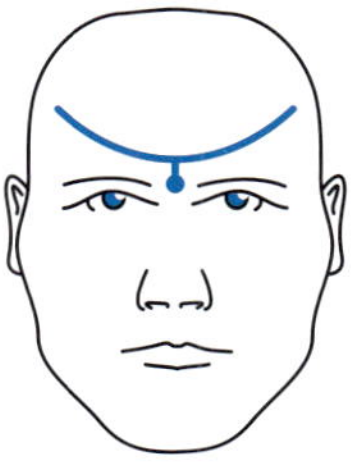

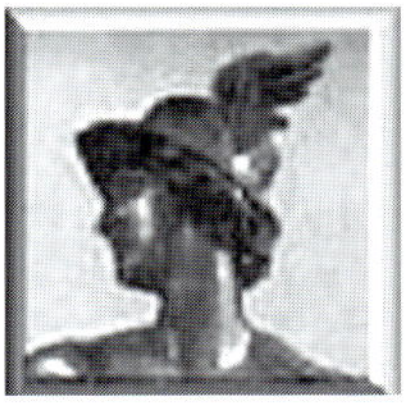

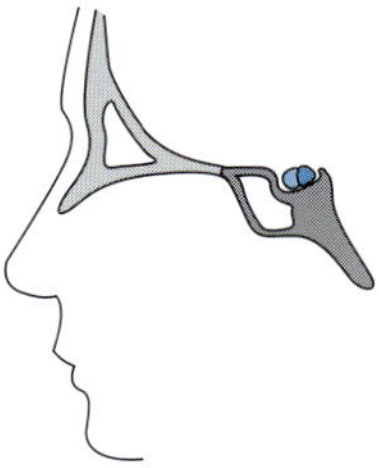

Mercury amalgams are a mere two centimeters away from the pituitary gland. Vapor from these amalgams has an affinity for this gland in high concentrations. The effect of these vapors on this gland can bring about hormonal disruptions and menstrual cycle disorders.

The fetal pituitary gland – which affects development of the endocrine, immune and reproductive systems – concentrates mercury.

... research in Sweden had revealed that the pituitary glands of Swedish dentists contained 40 times the average level of mercury found in the general population. The article also mentioned that in the United States, 70% of dentists with elevated mercury levels suffer from depression, anxiety and insomnia.

From Fracastoro's 'Syphilis'

..."But the right-hand path will set you by the waters of the sacred river, waters flowing with silver and living metal from which you can expect salvation.' And now they approached the golden halls and the mansions dripping with lead slag and caverns covered with streaks of black soot and grey sulphur. and now they were standing by wide swelling lakes flowing with quicksilver where they kept to the bank. 'Here is the relief found for your great toils,' continued Lipare. 'After you have been steeped three times in the living stream you will leave all this corruption behind in the sacred waters.' As she spoke thrice she bathed him in the silver fount of salvation, thrice with her virgin hands she scooped the river water over his limbs, thrice cleansed the body of the youth in its entirety: he marvelled at the old dishonoured skin sloughed off, his frame stripped of its malignant stain and the plague left beneath the flood.

...The strange tale received belief and the infallible treatment made its way through all the nations: at first pig grease began to be mixed in the liquid silver, then resin from the Aorician turpentine tree and from the lofty larch was added.

...Don't consider it repulsive nor disgusting to smear and cover the whole body; by such means the disease is removed, and nothing could be more repulsive than it. Yet spare the head and avoid the soft parts before the heart. Then on top bind bandages tightly and fasten dressings made of tow; next put yourself in bed with many blankets, until you sweat and the filthy drops flow over your body. It will be enough for you to have repeated this for ten days. It will be hard: but whatever the treatment brings must be borne. Be bold in spirit. Salvation as she stands right on the threshold will give you sure signs: you will constantly see the filthy liquified excretions of the disease pouring from your lips in the dirty spittle and you will be amazed at the large stream of corrupt matter before your feet.

...to cleanse your body, purify your limbs and sanctify your members with lavender and sprays of marjoram and rosemary, with sacred vervain and sweet scented lilies.

Friedrich Hahnemann

Friedrich Hahnemann, the son of Samuel Hahnemann, was born in Dresden in November 1786. Delicate in health and afflicted with spinal curvature, he had great powers of intellect and was considered a genius, speaking Latin, Greek, French, English, Italian and Arabic. He had various other qualifications and was a good musician (he played guitar and piano). Yet Friedrich possessed some very peculiar habits. He dressed in a bizarre manner and would tear into town on a four horse open wagon. Though successful in medical practice, he had many enemies, mostly among his colleagues, who joined forces to launch a general attack against him. After being summoned by the Royal Sanitary Commission of Saxony he fled, leaving his wife and daughter to become a wanderer. He moved from Germany to Holland, then on to England, Scotland and Ireland. On his travels he was subject to many adventures, including nearly drowning at sea. When he finally wrote to his distressed parents, he would not send an address, merely stating that he was travelling. His infrequent letters were wild in appearance, written mostly in the corners with large empty spaces on the page. Hahnemann was greatly grieved by his son's behaviour and absence, eventually admitting he was insane. Sometime around 1830 Friedrich moved to the United States, after which he was never heard from again.

Wherever the young Hahnemann settled for a short while, he practised a very eccentric brand of homœopathy. He would dictate extremely precise and demanding instructions, which often seemed ridiculous and difficult to follow. If they were not strictly adhered to he would fly into a rage and refuse to treat the offending patient. Yet he achieved remarkable cures, which astounded all who came in contact with him.

Later reports of Friedrich Hahnemann were of a five-foot hunchback, who, though only forty, had the appearance of a sixty year old. He was described as quick and vivacious, extremely irritable and passionate in disposition. He walked around unshaven wearing an old dressing gown, and preached that society was degenerate and needed to return to primitive simplicity. His irritable and dictatorial manner caused many conflicts. He was subject to much ridicule, often being sued or chased out of town by cured patients who could not abide his manner.

The majority prove more successful by using quicksilver to loosen everything completely; there is a miraculous power implanted in it. Whether because it is its nature to take up cold and heat instantaneously, so that it quickly gathers our body heat to itself and, because it is very concentrated, it breaks up the humors and acts on them with greater force, just as a white-hot flame makes iron glow more fiercely. Or the fierce particles, from which mercury with its marvellous structure is formed, are loosened from their own internal bonds and connections and, now able to be carried separately into the body, they melt the concretions and burn out the seeds of the plague."

Friedrich Hahnemann was last seen during the cholera epidemic of Northwest U.S.A. An eccentric German hunchback appeared in the lead mines of Galena, miraculously curing hundreds of people from a small vial that had neither taste nor smell. He asked no fees for his services.

His main writing was a 'Refutation of Hecker's Attack on the Organon of Homœopathic Healing by Samuel Hahnemann'. He participated in many of his father's provings, including Belladonna, Bismuth, Guaiacum, North Magnet, Staphysagria, Thuja and Mercury.

Phytolacca

"This is a very imperfectly proved remedy, and it is only possible to present fragments of it. The mental symptoms have not been brought out, but the remedy has some striking features."

"Phytolacca ought to be called "vegetable Mercury" because it is so full of symptoms analogous to Mercury."

Kent, *Lectures on Materia Medica*, 'Phytolacca'

Proving Of Phytolacca

Proving by female age 41
Took one dose of Phytolacca 30C
September 1997

NS – New symptom
OS – Old symptom
AS – Altered symptom
CS – Cured symptom
xx.xx.xx – day.hour.minute

MIND

Sensations – Body

05.08.xx My right side feels much more open than my left as though open for invasion, exposed.

07.xx.xx I feel split right down the middle, my left side feels much more substantial than my right. My right seems light, insubstantial, painless, easy to penetrate, from head right down to foot. My left side has various aches and pains, it feels more substantial, more tense, more compact. Aches in left head, shoulder, sacrum, thigh-front, calf, dorsum of foot. My left foot feels warmer than the right. The right foot is cold and a tingling is creeping up into the leg.

08.16.xx My body still feels split down the middle. But for once the left side of my head which is on the top feels light and it is my right which seems heavier, denser and tenser. So does all of my right side. My left feels lighter, less dense though the left-sided headache is still there.

08.17.xx During osteopathic treatment the split reversed again in that the left side became more dense and the right side lighter.

08.18.xx Now the right side is denser again and the left side lighter.

08.20.xx Split of body has reversed again, left side dense, right side light. It reminds me of alternating current. I am a metal after all.

08.22.xx Reversal again, left side light, right side dense.

09.07.xx My right side is quite insubstantial again while the left is dense.

09.18.xx My body is split into a dense left and a light right side.

10.xx.xx The split in the body is fainter now, right side full and left side empty.

11.xx.xx The left side of my body feels full and the right empty but there is no distinct split in the middle, rather the density diminishes gradually from left to right. In my mind's eye the left side of my body extends more, it bulges, while the right side is thin and drawn, reduced.

12.xx.xx Now it is the right side of my body which is full and extended, gradually turning into empty and diminished on the left side.

13.xx.xx Left side of body dense and extended, right side insubstantial and diminished.

15.xx.xx Left side of body dense, right side light.

16.xx.xx Left side of body slightly bigger and denser than the right.

17.xx.xx Right side of body feels more dense and bigger than the left.

18.xx.xx Left side of body more substantial and bigger than right.

19.xx.xx Left side of body feels very dense and enlarged while the right side is insubstantial and diminished.

Sensations – Head

00.00.19 My face feels distorted. The left eyebrow is much higher than the right which is pulled down. My face feels tilted to the right though I am holding my face straight as normally. The chin seems to be pulled towards the left shoulder. This continued all day.

04.22.xx Facial distortion still there, chin pulled to the left, right eye lower than the left.

05.08.xx My chin feels insubstantial on the right but more pronounced firm and substantial on the left.

07.08.xx I seem to have got used to the feeling of the displacement of my face. I notice it clearly when I concentrate but forget about it otherwise. My left side of head is on top and it is painful. The right side hangs down.

08.16.xx My right eyebrow seems to be pulled down over the eye like a cap. I see my chin in my mind's eye sticking out to the left but of light substance. My right jaw seems to hang down.

09.07.xx My facial distortion feels very pronounced as though the right side of face (and head) is light, insubstantial and smaller than the left which lies over the top with the chin sticking out to the left. What has changed is that the split seems not to involve the frontal lobes. Both are heavy and connected.

09.08.xx My head and face feel like this: the head is tilted to the right so that the left side of my head is on top and occupies about 80% of the mass while the right side is below and occupies only about 20%.

12.xx.xx My head feels strange. The distortion continues but the large overpowering portion on the left is light and insubstantial, the little portion on the right, particularly my right chin, feels like a very condensed, solid area which also seems to pull the right corner of my mouth downward in a kind of contraction with its centre in the right side of the chin. My right lower lip feels a bit numb.

13.xx.xx Distortion of face continues, left chin feels pulled to the left, right chin feels diminished. A tension pulling the right corner of my mouth downward (nothing can be observed).

16.xx.xx In my mind's eye the left side of my head and face is totally overpowering the right of which there is only the wing of the nose and a little bit of the cheek and chin.

17.xx.xx Left side of head feels lighter than right as though the head gets denser and denser from left to right. It still feels as though tilted to the right with the chin sticking out to the left. The left side has totally taken over and covered the right side as well as though a cover has been pulled over the face from left to right and is now being knotted at the right cheek/jaw.

18.xx.xx My head has only got a left side which is overpowering and heavy, getting lighter towards the right which is only an anatomical location or position. The right half of my head does not exist as an entity. The chin still feels like it is sticking out to the left.

19.xx.xx My head feels tilted to the right, chin sticking out to the left, with only the left side of the head existing. At the moment I also have the desire to physically tilt my head to the right.

24.xx.xx Left side of head seems larger than the right without, however, impinging on the right. I have both sides of my head back. There seems to be a clear split. The chin still points to the left but the head seems to be straightening out.

Delusions – General

03.02.50 Knowing with certainty that nobody else is in the house I nevertheless look suspiciously around me. I feel a presence, not actually human, and not very friendly. Invoked the good forces. Feel a bit spooky. Have to control myself not to search the whole flat. I check the phone to make sure there is a dialling tone. (AS – I do sometimes feel not totally alone and have looked behind me when walking upstairs in the darkness but this time it has happened with the lights on).

03.22.45 Doing some meditation after exercises I feel the malevolent presence again, very spooky. It comes from the right and seems to surround my right side from right back to all of my front as I am standing with closed eyes. It definitely feels like a circumscribed being or energy which seems to move with a purpose. I have been known to feel spooked when alone in the dark but not while engaged in my usual activities and while there is light. Again I have to invoke all the good and helpful forces. This energy seems to try and penetrate into me, dissolving my hands.

07.21.xx I am getting very distinct inner messages when I am not supposed to do any particular thing or when I should stop doing something. (AS – stronger than usual).

Delusions – Hearing

00.00.01 I hear a bell ringing the midnight hour (proving started at midnight). I have never heard a bell from my house before. It is fading in and out like carried by a gust of wind. There is no church near my house. The next church is more than half a mile away.

Grace, Gratefulness

00.00.32 Intense feeling of gratefulness to the universe for homeopathy.

19.xx.xx I have brief moments when I feel in a state of grace, grateful for doing the proving of this remedy. I feel as though some internal barrier has been broken down.

Playfulness, Humor

00.13.xx Very giggly, joking, singing, playing about, fooling about (AS – not usually with such abandon or to such a degree).

04.16.xx I am feeling a kind of hysterical giggle bubble up in my throat, desire to giggle.

05.12.xx A giggle bubbling up.

08.11.xx Feeling a bit hysterical, desire to giggle.

08.17.xx I had a real attack of giggles and laughter from my abdomen during the osteopathic treatment and had to control myself so I would stop. Just thinking about it makes me laugh again.

15.xx.xx Once in a while suddenly my humour breaks through and I can't help myself coming out with some flippant remarks, e.g. when exchanging notes with my supervisor. It is as though suddenly I am struck with something being hilarious or outright funny and despite feeling like death one minute suddenly have to chuckle at something or make light of it.

19.xx.xx I am able to chuckle at some things again. An irresistible giggle rises up from my abdomen at times without any apparent reason at all. It feels good though a bit embarrassing being in public. It is the flip side of crying which I could do nearly as easily.

25.xx.xx Still get these laughs coming up from nowhere for no reason.

27.xx.xx Every so often I start chuckling, the oddest things strike me as funny. Sometimes I laugh without an apparent reason.

Gloom, Depression, Weepiness, Thoughts of Death, Suicidal

06.17.xx I am very aware of the transitoriness and fragility of human existence. It is both an optimistic and a pessimistic thought. Optimistic because in the greater scheme of things what I do is really not very important, pessimistic because it warrants the question why I should make any effort at all. I have felt gloomy this afternoon but now this thought cheers me because it is really all about making this moment count, doing the right thing now whatever that may be. I could be dead and gone tomorrow, so what meaning would any plans have if I did not live while I was alive.

07.22.xx Sleep feels like a welcome escape, I have been looking forward to going to go to sleep the last few days and not only because I am tired. It is a good feeling, sinking into the oblivion. (OS – when depressed I used sleep as an escape some 15 years ago).

12.xx.xx I am in my dark side (OS/AS – I used to have depression 15 years ago).

13.xx.xx Very upset, I feel locked in depression, heavy, can't release any feeling, carrying on as though my feelings did not exist. It is as though my vital energy has been drained, immense sadness, washing over me like waves, like a black force of despair and loneliness. Desire to run away and hide, casting around in my mind what to do to snap out of this state. Antidote? Bach flowers? > talking about it and being listened to, > occupation, > eating a couple of mouthfuls of food. Extremely melancholy, locked in myself, how to break out? A physical feeling of wanting to tear my own skin off my body to break out of the prison of my body. Waves of despair attacking me. Fear of the state of total blackness. My insides are churning.

14.xx.xx I am starting to get obsessed with the idea that if I could only cry this would get better, I would feel better. I have a desire to scream to let out the raging heat. I have been depressed in the past, however never as intensely. The proving seems to amplify everything. I am worried how I will cope with normal life after this weekend. I am scared. What is happening to me? My insides are churning, I feel weak and tremulous. I am trying to ride the waves of despair, just stay with it. I feel on the verge of tears constantly but there is nothing I can do to release them or myself. Inconsolable. I am getting fed up with myself, feeling like a whinge. It is easier to pretend to the outside world if not to myself that none of this is happening. > talking about it.

I am scared to go to bed – just being overwhelmed by the feeling. At 5pm I got to a point where I just felt suicidal about it – nothing made sense, there is no point in being here. I hadn't really thought about how to go about it. I actually feel better when I've talked about it.

I can shut myself off while doing mental work, that is how I survive. I just wanted to go to some lonely place and scream, I'm scared it is never going to stop. Coping strategies just work for a short time and then I have to try something else. – Then I think maybe this is the opportunity of my life to face my demons – use anything to try to make sense of it. < from being alone. Being alone is freaking me. When I am in company it is easier to split it off. When I am on my own I can't. Scared of being overwhelmed, like being imprisoned, like being in a small room with something that's too big for the room and I can't get out. Last few days I am like somebody wildly banging against the walls and the less the walls give way the more I panic. I've never felt like this before. I have felt similar but less intense. It really feels like the darkest part of the night and it will never be day again. The difficulty is trying to explain it but I can't think of a reason. If the aggravation is this bad I hope the cure is much better.

15.xx.xx I feel awful, no light anywhere. I feel paralysed internally, don't know which way to turn to get relief, on the verge of tears but too weak to even try to release them. I feel awful dumping all this stuff onto my supervisor, keep pretending some normality while around her. When she left the house what happened felt symbolic because rather than waiting till she had gone to her car I shut the door. It was like shutting her out. It is awful. I feel mortified about myself. Why can't I get a grip? How can I expose anybody to the way I feel? I can't even let myself go when I am alone, I am afraid I would fall into a bottomless hole with no end. Isn't prison better?

Felt > after shedding some tears, > occupation, so my job may yet prove to be my salvation. I want to cry and cry and cry. The tears are coming ever closer to the surface. I am also feeling some anger rise up, I want to shake this enemy off. Get off my back! I want to scream, tear at my upper back, tear it off me.

I am sitting on a train and the only conversation I hear is somebody talking about prisons.

My reaction to food seems to be the same as my reaction to support. Both are nourishing and I feel better for them but it is very difficult to swallow them. As soon as I am given some support I feel that I don't deserve it. By asking I impose and will be abandoned. Once I start giving in to the crying I am going to be lost in endless blackness, dark and horrifying, I can't let anybody see it lest they desert me and leave me alone in this blackness. Memories of a childhood trauma are surfacing. (NS – I have never been aware of it or felt it like this before).

Suicidal. No sense in anything, there is no hope. I just want to lie down and become unconscious. > talking to people or being around people, more vulnerable when alone.

16.xx.xx No desire to get up. Fed up with the constant weakness, I feel as though beset by a parasite which is sucking all my energy out of me. Had to call into work sick. When getting ready to go to work this scream started building up inside my chest. Went back to bed and had a scream, then a cry. I want to find a place where I can sit in total blackness.

Light disturbs my eyes at the moment.

Memories of early childhood. Crying. The gloom is not lifting. I am getting fed up. Everything senseless, what is the use anyhow? No energy or will to tidy up (I am usually very fastidious and can't live in a mess!)

I want to let rip, scream, tear things up and go totally wild with rage. I want to face an enemy who is tangible, who I can fight. I want to do a sword fight and stab him with a loud scream. Alternating between misery and fury, feeling weepy and angry, angry and fed-up with myself.

I don't care whether I live or die. Had a cry but it seems to deepen the distress, not alleviate it. > talking to somebody, > when distracted by patients calling up.

17.xx.xx I feel weepy and helpless, fragile, not with it. Work feels meaningless. Very gloomy, no joy or spark in life, I feel awful though pretending normality at work. I feel like a person grieving. It is very difficult to discipline myself to stay at work. I don't dare leave the office for a lunch break because I may not find the energy or will to come back. I feel very much on edge, as though I am having some kind of breakdown. I am doing a pretty good job at keeping up pretences though it is difficult, nobody at work seems to find anything out of the ordinary. Difficult to be with people, exhausting, yet cannot stay alone for too long. Feeling of futility, coping with a moment at a time.

21.xx.xx Suicidal thoughts of drowning.

22.xx.xx Life feels totally devoid of joy; dull, two-dimensional, bleak.

25.xx.xx Bleak state of mind. Depressed even in a room full of people. Weepy and slightly nauseous. Everything seems empty and futile. I am tired of being vulnerable, depressed and needy, everything hurts me. Whatever strategy I apply, it does not work. > talking to friends.

I've had suicidal thoughts yesterday, the idea was of razor blades, first in the morning then in the evening. When I first woke up I wanted to disappear, to fall into blackness and not to feel anything and since that doesn't happen spontaneously one has to lose a bit of blood. I try to hold very still – I try to let the thought be there and then I try to help myself give comfort or whatever and talk to myself. The same in the evening before I slept. Today I am just incredibly sad.

30.xx.xx In half-sleep and when waking the depression came over me again. Weepiness. It is a nearly physical sensation of a cloud enveloping me. > from being held and cuddled.

32.xx.xx Slight cloud of depression with weepiness on waking, > being hugged.

33.xx.xx I feel more and more normal and myself, as though something that had taken me over is withdrawing from my system, like an insidious invader. While it was happening I was not aware of it as strongly as now when it is leaving me. Suddenly I remember who I am, I feel familiar to myself, I recognize traits within myself coming back, such as motivation, drive, conscientiousness, the tendency to meet challenges head-on.

Sensitivity, Alternating Moods

00.09.15 Worried that I haven't expressed myself correctly during the case taking prior to the proving and that some things might be misconstrued or misunderstood, particularly that I may be judged as unfeeling, cold or frigid for saying that I hardly ever cry or that I am very rarely interested in sex. (AS – I tend to worry about what people think about me but not as concretely as this nor for these issues.)

00.xx.xx I feel tumultuous emotionally. Changeable, up, down, sideward. Annoyed one minute, sad and weepy the next, then again in hysterics, very emotional. Feelings are flying through the air, I don't know what to do with them.

01.06.45 Woke up grumpy, in a bad mood (AS – not usually on waking).

05.xx.xx I am feeling a bit volatile today, sensitive to what others say. In the morning I made some remark about how nice it would be to be outside (the sun was shining and it was beautiful outside) and not to have to be in the office. One of my team members then said that I had the wrong profession. So I kept on the banter by saying, maybe I should have become a gardener whereupon she said, no, the Queen because the Queen could do what she wanted (which isn't true) but I felt a bit offended and hurt wondering whether I am ruling over my team and whether that has prompted the remark. It took a while to let it go, anyway I just shut up and did not continue the discussion but felt bad for a while. (AS – I am usually quite sensitive but not so acutely).

09.23.xx Feeling weepy since talking to my supervisor. Felt not taken seriously and respected by her when she chuckled while taking my symptoms. Though I am sensitive at the best of times I usually protect myself better. I seem to be more open and vulnerable than usual. (AS).

10.04.xx Still thinking of the incident on the phone last night, can't go back to sleep.

10.07.xx I recognise now that I have had mood swings over the last few days which seem to be sudden. One minute I feel nearly ecstatic, the next I can feel very upset and close to tears. Both seem to be aspects of the same heightened sensitivity.

10.21.xx Feeling very fragile emotionally.

11.06.xx Weepy and on the edge of tears but cannot release them (AS – usually I can make myself cry with some effort).

11.08.xx My headache is better (I always have a headache when I suppress tears). I lay down in bed quietly for a while after waking up and willed the energy of my unshed tears to come down from my head into my chest and abdomen. I have never done this before nor even had the idea to do so. Now I feel more peaceful and positive.

11.20.xx After feeling quite good and positive in the morning I had a meeting with a colleague who was quite antagonistic and aggressive. I felt a bit battered and very sensitive. I wonder whether I am cut out for my job. I need a lot of reassurance at the moment, cannot handle antagonism of people even if not directed against me personally.

12.xx.xx I need a lot of reassurance. Very upset about my colleague who got sacked. Fragile emotionally.

18.xx.xx Extremely grumpy on waking (AS). Can't find the energy to cheer up. Screaming and crying, I feel locked in my misery, nobody can help me, if only I could make a connection. I feel like a wounded animal in its lair, lying curled up in my bed. I want to strike out and bite, stick my claws into somebody. Biting my own lips. I am so alone. I want a cuddle! Every so often an overpowering desire to scream. It is really frustrating not to be able just to do it (I am at work).

I keep on talking to myself, to the things around me. No strength to 'behave' normally. I am not rational or composed. Feel like a slightly deranged person, the ones seen in the street sometimes, muttering to themselves, carrying on in their own world, oblivious of the expectation of normality or perhaps just ignoring it.

I try to avoid thinking because when I do the sense of futility overpowers me. I can't think ahead, can't look forward to anything. I have to stay right where I am at the moment. > mental occupation, it makes me unaware of my feelings.

19.xx.xx Crying and screaming > talking to people, mental occupation. < physical occupation because it makes me think.

21.xx.xx Up and down every minute – sometimes laughing, sometimes crying, mostly crying.

22.xx.xx Very grumpy on waking.

I want to get angry at people, am looking for reasons to get angry at them. I'd like to blame somebody but there is nobody to blame. I want to get at somebody for the way I have felt and am still feeling. Weepy and crying. I am fed up! I don't want to cooperate anymore. Helplessly furious.

I feel humiliated for being such a whinge. I cannot trust people to be honest with me because they'll make allowances for the 'proving'. But what do they really think about me? If they had a choice, wouldn't they be running a thousand miles? Total lack of motivation, sense of futility, all seems senseless, I cannot even think one minute ahead.

23.xx.xx I feel delicate and weepy.

25.xx.xx I'm not irritable. Usually, when everything gets up my nose I want to snap. I haven't had any of this. I'm incredibly laid back, I take care of myself, sit in the hammock for hours listening to music.

27.xx.xx Bleak mood, as though there is no future. Nothing to look forward to. Just existing in this moment, no joy, no sorrow.

41.xx.xx I feel exasperated about yet another friend of mine being sacked from her job.

Separation Issues, Loneliness, Abandonment, Company, Touch

00.09.20 I really miss J. We both travel quite a lot and don't see each other for a week or two at a time. J. has only been gone for a couple of days but I feel as though part of my energetic body has been taken all the way to Shanghai. I feel like a magnet that is usually compact but now one pole has been far removed from the other and the bit in the middle has been stretched very taut.

03.xx.xx My general feeling tonight and yesterday has been sombre, a bit lonely and at loose ends. It is very difficult to actually do the things that need doing, I'd much rather just sit about moping.

05.xx.xx I have tried to arrange various meetings with different people for the weekend but have not been able to get through to anybody. I am inclined to give up, after all I left messages and nobody has got back to me. It should be good to be on my own and just be.

06.13.xx I feel upset, I want some cuddles, weepy.

07.08.xx I feel lonely, I definitely have greater difficulty with J's absence than usual. I feel like a whiny child that wants attention, desire to be cuddled and held, desire to whine and complain. No initiative to act maturely or make myself feel better. I want to just flop and let or have somebody else make it ok and make me feel better. I want somebody around me who can be my mother but I don't want anybody's company in front of whom I have to behave in a mature way. I feel totally selfish, I want to be making all the demands, I don't want anybody making any demands on me. > occupation, < thinking about it.

08.18.xx The osteopathic treatment wasn't cuddles but still I enjoyed the touch.

09.08.xx Desire for physical intimacy and affection (AS – usually not as aware of this nor is it as intense).

09.18.xx I want a cuddle.

10.06.xx I want to be cuddled and held.

11.xx.xx Desire for hugs and cuddles.

12.xx.xx Desire to be looked after, not taking the initiative, just drifting

13.xx.xx I don't know what to do with myself, I feel very alone, locked within myself. Could not force myself to write anything all day. Great need to be cared for and looked after which I felt >. Desire to be held.

14.xx.xx I am scared. What is happening to me?

17.xx.xx I feel awful, need to speak to someone. Tried to call people, could not reach anyone. > acknowledging to myself and writing down how I am feeling as though I am my own empathetic listener.

18.xx.xx I feel helpless. I want somebody to take it all away. I want somebody to hold me and reassure me. Very insecure, easily worried, I easily feel abandoned when I am not able to contact somebody. Need a lot of reassurance, feeling lost.

19.xx.xx Weepy on waking. I feel very alone. Upset and anxious when I cannot contact somebody.

I have been talking on the phone for most of the day.

20.xx.xx I feel very young, want to be looked after, unable to make decisions or initiative, being responsible. I need one-to-one attention, difficult to be in a large group, a state of selfishness, the needs of a small child. It is a struggle to give out anything. I don't feel like an adult. I feel like in my own world, grateful when people make contact with me but have difficulty to sustain contact with them, very turned on to myself. I want cuddles, physical affection, being stroked, body work. The feeling of loneliness is inconsolable, I can't break out of it. I feel like an infant, my movements seem to be limited. People drift into and out of my field of vision. It is up to them to make contact with me, I am helpless, I can't initiate the contact, I can't bring them into my world, I am alone, how can I bear it? > talking about it and being listened to empathetically by somebody who understands. Nobody can alleviate this loneliness.

21.xx.xx Lonely, crying, feeling abandoned, there is no way out. Why does nobody help me? Can anybody help me?

Angry, I want to tear the skin off my body, desire to scream. Desire to jump out of my skin. Very melancholy. Screaming, crying, laughing. I want to put my fist through a window, I am feeling myself going off the rails. Raging against my feelings, against everybody. I feel humiliated and shamed by the state I am in, I hurt so, I want to hurt somebody else, make them understand how it feels, take revenge for all I am going through, punish somebody, I don't want to co-operate any longer.

I am fed up with co-operating. Here I am laying myself open to scrutiny, revealing feelings that make me cringe, and what for? To feel what I have always feared most – that I am a nuisance, a burden and a liability. That's just great! For whom am I doing this bloody proving anyway? And then I should apologise for it, for being off my head? Oh yes, being the nice, considerate person I am, I bend over backwards apologising, trying to make things easy, trying to pretend I am normal, trying to be REASONABLE! Panicking that I might inconvenience anybody. Hell, what about my own inconvenience? Aren't we all in this together by mutual agreement? We all made an uninformed decision with this proving, not having a clue what could happen. But now that it has happened, I am supposed to deal with it all on my own?

The emotional pain is better from touching the middle of my sternum with my fingers and transmitting love energy through my fingers. It comforts me. I don't feel as black, as despaired but it's a more defined feeling, the real issue doesn't get resolved, the abandonment, utter loneliness. I try to devise all sorts of strategies to focus it – but I am not getting anywhere very fast – more difficult when I am with people. I feel tortured because life just goes on and they have their own stuff and it doesn't really matter whether I'm there or not.

Sometimes on my own I feel alone already, so I shouldn't be disappointed. but that doesn't really work either. What has been most helpful was talking to Silvie and what she said was "I don't want you to go". To get 100% attention, it felt like mirroring/homœopathic. It's not the same if I feel I am only getting divided attention.

22.xx.xx I want to go and hide, I want to break out, smash something, kick the walls down.

I switched on the radio – a radio play about prison.

23.xx.xx Melancholy when on my own, at loose ends. I need company. I feel easily deserted.

24.xx.xx I feel lonely and weepy and in pain. Trying to convince myself that I am surrounded by people who love me as I am but it is not enough. I need somebody with me, to hold me, to stay with me. I use music as my company. Not a whole orchestra, I want one melody, one instrument to speak to me, to be with me. Why is nobody listening?

Crying myself to sleep.

25.xx.xx The pain seems to be eating away at the inside of my chest. Nothing seems to shift it, it goes on and on. I am on my own.

27.xx.xx J. is back from Shanghai. We could not connect instantly. She is full of her experience, I am in my own world.

28.xx.xx J. and I have started to connect. It feels as though my aura is coming back together again. Strange feeling – quite a physical sensation like the rubber band which had been stretched so tight had come back – the front of my body – as if the front part of my body was missing. I feel more ... imagine you're a dumpling – ragged edges torn apart and now coming together like a cloud of energy torn in half and now joined up again.

34.xx.xx Still having difficulty to be on my own for long, > somebody around. Easily feel lonely.

Concentration, Efficiency, Motivation

02.xx.xx Concentration seems poorer than normal. I feel slightly spaced out, can't distinguish whether I can't or don't want to focus. I can't be bothered.

I am a little careless, can't be bothered to write legibly. Can't be bothered to explain details here. Much more content to explain it to my supervisor and let her write it down.

03.12.xx My motivation to work, i.e. sitting in front of a VDU, in an office, without moving much, is at an all- time low. I want to go home and be doing nothing. Preferably I want to have a nap.

03.18.xx Immense relief to be home after wishing all afternoon that I could go home.

04.11.xx Very unproductive at work, messing about.

04.12.30 My computer lost a document and has been playing up generally. Having lost the last 10 minutes of work was just the last straw. I am cursing and have thrown something against the screen. Stupid bloody machine!

04.13.15 Not my day today. Went to the hairdresser who cut my hair wrong. Is it me expressing myself wrongly? I thought I was so clear in what I wanted and how I said it.

05.07.xx No motivation to go to work.

05.22.xx I can't believe it! I missed one train by a few seconds shortly after 9pm. Had to take a different route than planned. Had to change my route again due to a security alert and missed another train by a few seconds. Took 2 hours for a journey of one. I seem to be repeating the phrase 'I can't believe it' frequently.

05.22.xx I still find it more comfortable to explain things in more detail to my supervisor rather than write them myself.

06.08.xx Just lying around. Part of me is happy to be doing nothing, the other is aware that quite a few things need doing.

06.13.xx I have been trying to work on a case for hours. Can't make head or tail of it though the case is clear. Can't find rubrics, can't pin the case down, can't stick to a train of thought. Jumping from one aspect to another, unproductive. Frustrated. I wish I could just finish the case and get it off my chest. Very aware that the patient is waiting for the remedy. If I had the choice I would just forget about it, but feel I don't have the choice. (Usually I am very systematic and patient). I can't go about the case in a systematic way, haven't got the staying power to do it.

06.14.xx I have decided on a remedy. What an intense relief this is! (AS – relief more than usual).

07.08.xx I feel grouchy. I don't want to do anything yet can't find the peace to just be. Then start doing something and find myself unmotivated.

08.07.20 It is a real struggle with myself to get up and get going. It has taken me close to an hour.

08.16.xx Very glad to leave work early to go to my osteopath. I am totally unmotivated at work and unlike usual I can't just ignore that and push myself. Very very glad to get out of there. I am only interested in doing exactly what I want to do. If it were not for the time it takes to get out of London I'd be out on a long walk. I find myself taking longer to do things. No energy to speed myself up.

17.xx.xx Cannot concentrate, cannot remember words.

18.xx.xx For the first time I've had a positive feeling that I could leave my job and something else would come up. I have thought concretely about the possibility of just walking out. What am I doing here?

20.xx.xx No interest in anything intellectual, can't make an intellectual effort. I want to do my own thing in my own time.

22.xx.xx No drive, no energy, no purpose. I cannot stay with anything for long. I want to be oblivious, not think, not feel. I cannot concentrate. Trying to keep myself occupied with little things.

23.xx.xx I seem to be better when engaging with people, having meetings. Normally meetings bore me to tears because of the slow progress. Today they seemed to suit my mental speed. I am not good at doing a lot of concentrated work right now. I am getting hardly anything done at all.
No staying power, nothing can hold my attention for long.

25.xx.xx Had a course at work all day today. It usually drives me 'round the bend', they're so slow. Today no desire to gallop ahead at all.

28.xx.xx Total lack of usual energy, drive and motivation. Not very active physically, hardly at all mentally. No stamina, easily discouraged. Everything seems too much, I can only cope moment to moment, can't plan or look to the future.

Memory

00.12.30 We went to visit Kew Gardens and I have forgotten the tickets for everybody. I can't believe myself!

01.08.xx I have forgotten to activate the answer-phone. I seem to forget things on the slightest distraction or when I multi-task. I start something or think of doing something, then get distracted and forget to go back to the task I have started.

04.06.45 Went to sleep last night thinking of a couple of things I should write. Now I can't remember a thing.

06.xx.xx My short-term memory is still very bad, I forgot to write this over the last few days but it happened on many occasions that I would start doing something or saying something and if not allowed to finish due to a distraction I would lose my train of thought or leave something unfinished. It would be impossible to find my train of thought again unless I made great efforts or when talking around the subject for a while. I would find uncompleted work after a while and then finish it.

12.xx.xx Blast! I have forgotten again to put the answer-phone on. I can't believe it! I have forgotten to bring my toothbrush.

Music

04.11.xx I want to listen to music, do my own thing.

09.23.xx I seem to be prepared to listen to only certain types of music the last few days. I have tried to listen to music that I usually like but it does not do anything for me. I mostly listen to Indian classical music and it makes me feel good.

10.xx.xx > from Indian classical music, being kind to myself, going about things quietly, not rushing or pushing.

15.xx.xx Finally able to cry a bit listening to Indian classical music. But it makes me feel suicidal.

20.xx.xx I need music to keep me going, Indian classical music, jazz. I can only listen to music with a single melody and percussion, cannot bear harmonies.

21.xx.xx Better from music as described but cannot bear TV, films, radio.

23.xx.xx Great desire for music, taking a walkman along everywhere, listening to jazz.

27.xx.xx I need music constantly but only solo instruments, Indian classical music, jazz, meditative music like Japanese or Sufi flute.

Language, Speech

00.11.30 My voice sounds louder to myself.

01.06.45 I am groaning and sighing a lot to myself.

02.07.45 Groaning and sighing to myself.

05.12.xx I feel I have talked too much and too loudly all morning. I am told by a friend that I am more talkative than usual.

19.xx.xx Talking to a friend on the phone I spoke Spanish fluently (usually I can only do so haltingly). She remarked on it.

23.xx.xx Groaning and moaning.

Time

03.08.xx I cannot rush myself. Have to do things in my own speed and time which is slower than usual. I noticed the same yesterday. Nearly missed a train, ran for it and got it in the nick of time.

06.13.xx Worried about time passing, I want to have some time for me!

07.10.xx I want to keep on jumping from one thing to another, there is not enough time to complete one thing before going to the next.

10.xx.xx There is no time for anything. I wish I did not have to go to work.

Invasion of identity

01.06.45 I am not myself but cannot describe how I am different.

31.xx.xx I feel suddenly I've re-emerged as though the remedy was a parasite, took over, invaded me etc. and has now beaten a retreat.

Things Falling, Coming Undone (anecdotal)

05.xx.xx Photos fixed to the wall with blue tack keep dropping to the floor throughout the proving.

05.16.xx A map which has been tacked to the wall in the office since I joined, 14 months ago fell off the wall for no reason.

06.23.xx Another photo has come off the wall, I can't even find it, I just noticed the gap.

12.xx.xx The colleague that I dreamed about got sacked today. I am very upset about it. The friend of a friend also got sacked today.

Jewellery

04.xx.xx I am wearing a little silver ring on the little finger of my left hand. I never wear rings as they give me bone pains. There is a little but bearable pain.

05.xx.xx Wearing the silver ring also today.

10.08.xx I am wearing a silver chain today. I don't usually wear jewellery and only gold when I do.

18.xx.xx Fussy about what jewellery I should wear. I cannot go near gold at the moment. (Jeremy said I should use Aur 30 to antidote if I need to).

Colours

00.09.30 I absolutely have to wear a light greenish turquoise cardigan I have worn a maximum of 3 times in as many years. Green socks as well.

01.08.xx I am wearing the same green/turquoise again as yesterday, and green socks.

03.xx.xx I don't like black though I am wearing it since many of my business clothes are black. I want muted greens, brown, nothing with red in it.

04.08.xx I have been able to wear hardly any black today, only my socks are black. Otherwise I am in green, brown and a little white.

04.08.xx When on the train going to work this woman sat down beside me who had huge fingernails painted in green with glitter in it, a nice green, rather like green olives. That's the colour I wear today as well.

18.xx.xx I hate black clothes. Fussy about what to wear.

DREAMS

00.xx.xx I suddenly realise that I am working for the Mafia while working in my current job. I see a man in black with a black hat talk to somebody at work. He represents the Mafia for me.

01.04.xx I am being mugged, held at knife point. I defend myself by biting. The muggers also have a dog that I wound mortally. I bite and then have to spit out the flesh I have torn out of my adversary's body.

I wake up two unconscious people by laying my hands on them and willing them to wake up. They get up as if nothing has happened.

Can only remember snippets of my dream – all about changing a room in a house (not mine) and a man who is so ill that he can only drink Coke for his food. I also remembered some of my Hebrew in the dream but have forgotten what it was now.

05.05.xx Trying to remember in my dreams what to write. Dream of arranging a room which was too cluttered, I wanted to clear it out, tidy it up.

10.04.xx Dreams of dead people.
I saw a woman lying at the bottom of a river. We brought her murderer to the scene of the crime.. I think he jumped into the water to try and escape.

I go to the memorial service of a person I know who is still very much alive in real life. We go to her house to say farewell to her and she is there herself but we all know she is dead. She just needs to say farewell to us all, then she disappears and one of her friends says that it was a great effort for her to appear to us in her body as though she is still alive.

11.06.xx I dreamed of having a meeting with work colleagues. Some of them kept on talking and disturbing the rest of us despite requests to stop.
One woman in particular kept on making a point of not co-operating to emphasise that she did not need to listen to us, we had no authority to tell her what to do. The meeting broke up without conclusion. I started arguing with her and ended up slapping her in the face once. I knew that she would retaliate. So I just stood there waiting until she was ready and then she slapped me on

my left cheek. After that I tried to keep on telling somebody what had happened because I felt bad about having lost my temper but was prevented constantly by other things going on.

12.07.xx I dreamed that I attended a seminar, I don't know about what, and none of the people there were known to me. It seemed to take place in a small village in quite basic facilities. Some of us were sitting on the floor in the lecture hall that was made of just cement and earth, some of it wet. At one point I went out and looked at myself in a mirror and got a shock. My forehead was very very high and the hairline drawn far back. There were many parallel lines on my forehead and my hair was a wild mane around my face.
I tried to straighten myself up and returned to the lecture. There was a deep, narrow box near the lecturer and an insect flew into it. The lecturer said to try and catch and kill it because this was A. Hitler and we would change the course of history. Several of us kept on trying to reach to the bottom of the box and catch or just kill the insect but nobody succeeded, it was too deep for our arms. At the same time the insect, which looked like nothing I have ever seen with an ivory white body shaped like a heart and many long legs and wings like a dragon fly, tried to escape repeatedly. Finally I placed a paper over the top of the box to wait until the insect would hold onto the paper. Instead it was strong enough to lift the paper a little and wiggle its way out on one side. One of its sides was damaged. Everybody told me to kill it quickly but I could not and it flew away before anybody else could catch it. So the terrible course of history remained unchanged. Then we all went to our respective rooms to break for lunch. I felt at loose ends and unsure what to do next.

19.xx.xx I dreamed that my father came to visit me (he has never ever done that). I had some kind of singing performance and when I saw him I was glad even though my singing was less than perfect. I forgot the words of my song at the end and stopped abruptly. But it didn't matter. He was old with the frailties of old age. I just felt affection and empathy for him.

20.07.xx Dreams of overthrowing governments, of planning assassinations, of being persecuted, of trying to break out from prison, of defending myself and a few others with any means at our disposal, of humiliating the enemy, of inventing strategic tricks to make an escape. e.g. I am shooting at enemy weapons which are placed to go off automatically when somebody gets into the line of fire, to make them go off prematurely. I spray an enemy political rally with yoghurt until the whole hall is wet and white. I escape but am caught with

2 or 3 others and while our captors prepare to kill us we scheme how to kill them by using any means we can find, e.g. driving a screwdriver into somebody's ear, offering to cut somebody's hair so that we can get at their throat, trying to trick our captors by flattering them, by appearing weak and helpless, by playing on their male vanity.

26.07.xx Dream of being healed by three women. The dream felt very good.

HEAD

00.00.05 Prickling movement on scalp.

00.00.14 Headache in right temple, eyebrow, forehead (AS – usually on left side).

00.23.xx Right-sided headache over eyebrow on lying down in bed (AS – usually left-sided headache).

01.20.xx Headache over right eyebrow. (AS).

02.09.45 Sudden stitching headache in left forehead for about one minute (AS – my headaches are usually dull).

09.07.xx Right-sided headache (AS).

10.14.xx Dull pressure building up in occiput and vertex (AS – dull pressure is usual but not in these locations).

16.xx.xx Right-sided headache. (AS).

17.xx.xx Right-sided headache – forehead (AS).

26.xx.xx Tearing, nervy pain on left side of my head above ear, lasted for about one hour (AS – I get lots of pain on the left side of the head but never tearing).

30.xx.xx My hair has suddenly grown very fast (noticed both by me and, independently, by a colleague).

31.xx.xx I have slept with two pillows throughout the proving and now have gone back to the usual one.

EYE

08.23.xx When opening my eyes after meditating for about 20 minutes my vision was totally blurred as if there was a film on my eyes. It took a few moments to clear through blinking and rubbing.

09.18.xx Sudden pain in right eye ball, for about a minute.

EAR

20.xx.xx Strong white noise in my ears on waking.

26.xx.xx Slight crackling sound in the ears as one hears when passing under pylons, on waking.

FACE

00.00.01 Heat rising from my neck to my face.

17.xx.xx Internal tremor in facial muscles.

24.xx.xx My left nostril has been solidly blocked on waking for a few days now. The left sinus seems to be totally blocked up as well and is somehow connected with the distortion of my face of which I am still aware.

MOUTH

00.05.00 Full and buzzy feeling in lips, more the lower than the upper.

00.11.00 Lower lip feels very warm and full, slightly buzzy.

03.23.30 As soon as I lie quietly in bed the buzzing in the lips, particularly lower, returns.

05.22.30 Severe itching on left side of tongue. It makes my eyes water.

06.08.xx Buzzing in lips, quite a voluptuous feeling.

07.08.xx Voluptuous feeling in lips. I want to be kissed.

07.22.xx Buzzing in lips, tingling.

08.23.xx Intense tingling in lips.

09.xx.xx Tingling and pulsating in lips.

09.18.xx Sudden burning in left side of tongue lasting for a couple of minutes.

09.xx.xx Still very aware of left side of tongue, the same place which itched intensely a few days ago, for 4 hours.

09.23.xx Intense buzzing in lips before sleep.

10.xx.xx Intense buzzing in lips < lower lip.

11.xx.xx Full feeling in lips, buzzing.

12.23.xx Buzzing in lips and upper front teeth, very intense, nearly a toothache.

16.xx.xx Sudden and very intense buzzing in the lips.

18.xx.xx Buzzing and tingling in lips. Buzzing in upper front teeth, nearly like a toothache.

19.xx.xx Intense buzzing in lips.

Stomach

07.xx.xx No appetite (AS – I can have that when emotionally upset but usually a very good eater).

09.xx.xx No appetite.

11.xx.xx Low appetite.

xx.xx.xx I have been off chocolate and without desire for it since the start of the proving. This is quite remarkable.

12.xx.xx No appetite but more thirsty than usual.

13.xx.xx Can eat only very little and have to struggle to keep the food down. Resistance to swallowing any solid or dry food. Desire for soft, juicy things.

15.xx.xx No appetite. I am forcing myself to eat but the food gets stuck in my throat and does not want to go down. It takes an effort to keep it down.

17.xx.xx Even more thirsty than usual (AS).

19.xx.xx No appetite, cannot eat at all.

20.xx.xx No appetite, can hardly eat at all, food sticks in my throat.

25.xx.xx Nauseous as soon as I eat even one bite too much.

27.xx.xx Very little appetite. Losing weight.

Abdomen

22.xx.xx Discomfort and flatulence for last 2 days, after mushrooms.

Stool

18.xx.xx Stool smells like a cow shed, after having some cheese.

Chest

01.15.xx Feeling in my chest as though my heart is weak.

13.xx.xx Burning in upper chest and back down to waistline.

14.xx.xx Burning in upper chest and back down to waistline intensified.

24.xx.xx Burning pain in upper chest.

Back

00.00.07 Pain in bottom end of right scapula.

04.13.15 With weakness in extremities felt an energy running up the upper part of my spine into the neck, like a charge, producing a slight shudder in the upper body. It is rather pleasurable, like the feeling of energy running up the spine during meditation.

04.22.xx My right back feels vulnerable.

16.xx.xx A current of energy running up my upper spine.

17.xx.xx Energy running up my upper spine making me shudder.

18.xx.xx Little thrills of energy running up my upper spine occasionally.

25.xx.xx Energy running up my spine making me shudder.

Extremities

00.00.05 Hands very warm.

00.00.32 Intense feeling and buzzing in palms of both hands.
Weakness in lower arms and legs, like a lack of substance, hollowness.

00.08.30 A kind of internal shaking in lower arms.

01.14.30 Weakness in arms, legs, as if I have done excessive exercise which I haven't, as if the muscles are trembling after a strong exertion but I haven't done any strenuous exercise.

02.18.xx Sore all over my back and arms after doing nothing different from normal, an internal trembling in the lower arm muscles as though over-exerted.

04.06.45 My hands and lower arms feel so weak I can hardly hold the pen, a kind of tremulousness felt in the muscles. The same in my legs and feet, to a lesser extent in my body. My fingers are a bit swollen, they look like sausages to me.

04.08.xx Feeling of total lack of strength and substance in my hands.

04.13.15 Sat at the hair dresser when the tremulous weakness came back in my arms, legs, abdomen. It feels as if there is no strength and substance.

04.23.30 Just before sleeping I had a sudden pain twice for a few moments in the front of my left thigh.

05.07.xx Fingers look slightly swollen again.

05.xx.xx Lack of strength in hands, when making a fist there seems to be a lack of substance.

05.14.xx Tremulousness in arms, < thinking about it.

05.23.30 Tremulous weakness in arms and legs while speaking about it.

07.08.xx The weakness and lack of substance, particularly in the hands seems to be stronger in the morning. I still cannot make a fist that gives me any feeling of strength.

07.xx.xx I have had a strange sort of cold feet in bed the last few days. Usually I have warm feet while I sleep. This morning I woke up with a feeling as of cold socks on my feet and the skin feels cool to the touch. This is different from cold feet where the cold seems to penetrate right through. My feet feel as though the skin around them is contracting, a bit of tingling with an unpleasant sensation of cold.

07.18.xx Tremulous weakness in lower arms and a bit all over after eating.

07.22.xx Sudden boring pain in my right hand between ring finger and little finger after writing for the last five minutes.

08.xx.xx Pain on left iliac crest while walking. I had it yesterday as well but forgot to write it.

08.xx.xx No strength in fists.

10.xx.xx Lack of strength in lower arms and hands.

12.xx.xx Woke up with severe tremulousness in my hands, very weak, > stretching. Weak legs.

14.xx.xx Intense weakness in lower arms and hands on waking.

16.xx.xx No strength in hands, fingers slightly swollen.

17.xx.xx Buzzing on surface of and weakness in lower arms and hands.

18.xx.xx Intense buzzing, nearly a tingling, high-pitched like an intense white noise, rather felt than heard in lower arms and hands, lower legs and feet. Sometimes crawling like ants.

19.xx.xx Intense buzzing in lower arms, hands, lower legs, feet, tingling.

23.xx.xx Feeling of cold socks on my feet on waking.

24.xx.xx Excruciating pain in my right leg on the outside of my right knee (I had that two years ago as well because I put my tibial-fibular joint out and had to punch it back into place). Also pain in the left leg this morning but less intense (never put the joint out in this leg).

25.xx.xx Pain in right tibial – fibular joint is so strong, I cannot bend my leg to more than a right angle.

26.xx.xx Sudden pain on inside of left knee, lasted for about one hour at the same time as the tearing headache.

27.xx.xx Severe pain in right foot during the night, could not find comfortable position, gone in the morning.

32.xx.xx Weakness in hands, as though my gripping power is not quite substantial.

Sleep

01.xx.xx Waking frequently in the early morning.

01.14.30 Very sleepy and tired – not due to eating since I had lunch at 12.00 (I can feel sleepy directly after lunch).

02.06.30 Can absolutely not get out of bed, very very sleepy.

02.14.xx Very sleepy in the afternoon. The whole body feels sleepy with desire to stretch but not > from stretching. (AS – usually >).

03.07.20 I overslept and still could go on sleeping. Very, very sleepy.

03.19.15 Whole body feels sleepy.

04.xx.xx Trying to wake up because thirsty but could not.

05.14.xx Very sleepy 2 hours after eating lunch.

08.06.xx Very sleepy on waking, can't really wake up, great resistance to doing so. It seems more important when I wake up than how many hours I have slept. More sleep does not >. Very difficult to find the will power to get up.

10.14.xx Very sleepy after eating. Very tired all day.

11.06.xx A new sleeping pattern has emerged: I go out like a light as soon as I lie down in the evening and seem to sleep very deeply till the early morning hours. It makes no difference how late I go to bed. Then I surface around 4 am – 5 am to spend the rest of the night in a kind of half-sleep filled with dreams not many of which I can remember.

13.xx.xx Same pattern as days 11 and 12. Struggling with being out of my body after waking from deep sleep at 5 am. Could not move beyond the room I sleep in. Made a supreme effort to awake and snapped back into my body at around 8 am.

Fever/Chill

00.04.10 Feeling hot lying on the right side, feeling chilly lying in the same spot on my left side.

01.06.45 Feeling hot lying on the right side, feeling cold internally when lying in the same spot on my left side.

04.22.xx Cold and shaky with icy cold hands.

25.xx.xx Very hot during the night. I threw a cover off even though there was frost outside and the window was open.

Skin

00.00.07 Itching on right middle finger. There is a raised pimple like a bite. I hadn't noticed it before. The pimple has a vesicular head.

Itching on right scalp, left earlobe, under left ear, around right ear, on right lower leg, on dorsum of left foot, on forehead, on right lower ribs.

00.00.13 Itching in small spots moving around the body surface. Continued for more than 4 hours.

00.23.xx Itching in spots wandering around the body after lying down in bed.

01.08.xx My skin seems to mend quickly. Yesterday I cut myself on paper. Not only did it not seem to hurt for so long but also the cut seemed to dry up quickly. The edges of the wound have not actually connected, but its surface is sealed and not painful. (CS).

02.11.xx A very small skin tag which I have had under my right eye for years seems to be getting very big and visible. It has been nearly invisible for 8 years but became even smaller after Thuja in May. Now it is big and rough (and continues to be after more than 7 weeks).

03.02.50 I was woken by intense itching in many little spots all over my body. Sometimes the itching intensifies into stinging. e.g. right cheek, right ear lobe, left axilla, right elbow, upper chest, left wrist, back of neck, genital area, left thigh, sole of left foot, inner left ear. Nothing visible on skin. It drives me nuts.

04.04.30 Woken up with very intense itching in various spots. Skin clear.

05.07.xx Woken earlier due to severe itching and pain in hands.

05.22.xx Itching all over the body in spots, left heel, between scapulae, right knee, upper abdomen, right upper eyelid, right lower eyelid, right side of right foot, right top of head, left temple.

06.08.xx Itching in spots again, left eyebrow, left lower arm, right jaw, left nostril.

24.xx.xx I've noticed that my skin is incredibly clear compared to normal. Last two days one spot close to the right axilla (unusual place!).

29.xx.xx Itching in spots all over the body, driving me nuts during the night. Some spots itched persistently for hours, e.g. inside of left wrist, right forehead, right wing of nose. Not > scratching.

41.xx.xx A wart I have had on the inside of my left big toe for months is now disappearing (CS).

GENERALITIES

01.12.10 Feeling of weakness and shaking in abdomen, arms, legs, as of 'nerves'.

01.15.20 I feel faint as if about to collapse. (AS – I used to get this sometimes after fasting without water for a day but never spontaneously).

02.19.xx Trembling in muscles continues, especially my arms, but also all over. Extremely tired.

03.02.50 I was lying on my right side when I woke up and my whole body felt as if a low voltage current was running through it, a definite sensation of buzzing in the skin and soft tissue, particularly in limbs and lips. The buzzing is more felt than heard and is more intense where skin meets skin, e.g. lips, inside of legs. I feel like a metal through which a current is passing. It is whitish, silvery.

04.16.xx Growing weakness in my limbs and abdominal area < when not occupied. It is becoming more and more like an internal buzzing similar to the noise one hears when passing under pylons, only I feel rather than hear it.

04.21.xx Feeling of weakness increasing in limbs and abdomen, as though I have fasted for a while or am being very dehydrated but I am drinking and eating normally. It is difficult to write, move or walk.

05.07.xx Whole body tremulous on waking.

05.xx.xx The feeling of weakness has receded a bit, it is less tremulous and more like a lack of substance, but it is there constantly.

05.17.xx Tremulous weakness < from thinking about it or when not occupied.

08.06.xx Weakness, particularly in limbs and chest on waking. Very tremulous, it feels as though my heart cannot cope.

08.13.xx Weakness all over after eating.

08.xx.xx I can feel my heartbeat rock my body when I am sitting.

09.xx.xx Weakness, most pronounced in lower arms and hands. Tiredness.

09.18.xx Felt like fainting while in the supermarket. A feeling like dehydration but I have had 2 litres of fluid today. Feeling weak and washed out.

12.xx.xx I can feel my heartbeat pulsing through my body while sitting. Feeling quite faint and weak sitting down after walking.

13.xx.xx Weight loss over the last few days.

14.xx.xx Intense buzzing in all of my upper body as though a current running through, I can nearly hear it, not only feel it < chest, upper back, lower arms and hands, on waking. My energetic body feels torn open < chest and upper back down to waist.

15.xx.xx Awful churning in my body on waking. Weak all over - arms, hands, abdomen, chest. Tremulousness and waves of burning passing over the surface of my body and upper back. My heartbeat is shaking my body, pulsating. Shaking in hands, my heart feels weak. My chest and abdomen feel hollow, my upper chest full of unshed tears. I am exhausted. Weak and ill with the emotional despair. No energy to do anything, no will either.

16.xx.xx Very weak. I can feel my pulse in every finger, all over the body. Buzzing on the surface of my body everywhere but < limbs and lips. I feel like in a state of suspended animation. Exhausted.

17.xx.xx The whole surface of my body is buzzing and tingling like from a low current. Weak and tremulous < lower arms and hands, my heart feels weak. I can feel my pulse in my eyelids when closing my eyes, heartbeat throughout the body. Buzzing in muscles. Weakness getting worse as day goes on. I feel totally shattered.

18.xx.xx My body feels like a live wire < lower arms and hands, nearly painful. Can feel heartbeat/pulse throughout my body. Very weak, tremulous. hollow feeling in abdomen and chest.

23.xx.xx Symptoms much stronger on waking than in the last few days. The whole body like a live wire, the buzzing is nearly a droning. Very weak feeling in the heart, weak all over, tremulousness, hands shaky, no strength in my grip, heartbeat shakes the body. I can feel my pulse to the last and outmost extension of my body, in the skin, the finger tips.

Symptoms as if developing a cold: Left nostril and sinus congested, sneezing, watery coryza. Rawness in larynx, hot and congested head, weakness, left-sided headache. Chilly and a bit feverish. All symptoms diminished after drinking some orange juice and water and totally disappeared by late afternoon (usually my colds last for at least a couple of days).

My osteopath remarked that my pulse can be felt into the smallest blood vessels, it is very pronounced.

25.xx.xx Woke at around 3 am with the most intense buzzing throughout my body yet. The voltage seems to be going up.

I cut my left index finger tip and could hardly stop the bleeding. I had to apply a pressure band aid and even then it kept on bleeding profusely for a while though the cut was not very deep.

32.xx.xx Occasional buzzing in body which seems to be connected to the heartbeat and pulse, it is stronger in the pause between the beats.

33.xx.xx Buzzing in single parts, it feels as if in one nerve, in one finger.

Phytolacca Blues

Delusion divided
one torn in two
what's left of me
had been right for you

Lonely winds sigh
tree bows its head
cloudy grey sadness
green turning red

And a single leaf falls
with nothing to say,
but long for the ending
of shortening days

Old book by your bedside
makeup unused
your smile not warming
my cool autumn blues

As my embers concede
to their fireplace death
I turn out the lights
and curl my cold bed

Delusion divided
one torn in two
and the empty space
that was left by you.

Phytolacca Synthesis

Verb

Sensation:
Divided, torn, split down the middle.

Function:
Must tilt to one side. Alternating.
Tilting to one side – dark or light, full or empty.
Alternating sides – Buzzing, current.

Noun

Silvery metal. Knife. Root.

Source:
Root – enveloped by black cloud.

Image

Blackness and bleakness alternating with giggle and grace.
Divided relationships, absent lover, dead mother.
One side empty - forsaken grief.
Empty side exposed to invasion by evil. Intangible enemy.
Lost in endless despair, darkest night, rage. Wounded animal. Prison.
Rebellion, assassination, subterfuge.
Vegetable Mercury, vegetable Platina.

Anecdotal Information

This information was presented to me be by Jake Kiakahi as an experimental project on 'inductive proving'. The remedy, Phytolacca 30C, was unknown to the prover and supervisor. The prover, who is highly sensitive, held the vial in his hand for approximately two hours. Due to the proving's unorthodox methodology, we present it as anecdotal information. It is up to each individual reader to use or disregard it. Time will tell if this information has validity.

O = Observation

O: He is scowling
A taste in mouth like a noxious liquid, like ammonia.
Anxious, a lot in the forehead.
Paranoid; "where are they?"
O: Hard shaking of legs
There's really strong fear.
O: Legs are jumping and spasming, he is breathing hard.
I'm wanting to check behind me. Frightful and freaking out.
It's fast, tremory, jittery.
Something like white or silver balls.

The sky and space are too big and threatening. Things don't feel in their proper place. As if the structure of the room isn't solid. It could shift really rapidly. Feels like a subway station where the trains are coming and going really fast, a white hall, reflections in the glass windows, silver cars that seem rickety.

There's a force coming at me, from behind. It's skewed.

Someone going crazy at a hospital. Paranoid. No orientation. I'm just watching things spin.
O: He is spinning in a swivel chair looking upwards toward ceiling.

Spaces and expansion. Like an Escher drawing, I can't tell what's what, like a cathedral from the inside. It's drug-like with the shapes changing.

The feeling is "the sky is falling, the sky is falling!"

There is something surreal, paranoid, and anxious, like a brain cry feeling, the frontal lobes of my brain are excruciating. I'm looking around quickly checking different areas. When I'm looking around quickly I can't fix on anything, everything is sort of surreal. Everything is interesting but scary too like it could drip away.

Things are unstable somehow. There's something about corners and arches. I feel taller. My height is funny. It's like being in a funhouse. A change in perspective; I can't get my balance right.

A cold-blooded white fright.

There's a scene in Exorcist III. There's a hospital ward with white coats. There's this possessed nurse (who attacks someone from behind). Metal going into my neck, like my head could be cut off. I'm checking behind me like something could come at me really quickly.
If I cried it would be in a laughing crying way. Very psychotic. A desire to scratch my head and bore in my nose. A lot of gestures.

O: He goes to observe a house fly in the window. He cautiously backs away from it.
It's not exactly fear. I'm fascinated. The instability of it I don't like.

O: He backs out of the room and hides behind the door in a dark hall.
I want to be sensorialy deprived.

There's a lot of fear. It's like a Hitchcock film when the camera zooms in on a doorknob and the doorknob has some significance. Drama, surreal, danger, fright, instability. But there is also a curiosity about stuff. I'm curious to go into the closet but I'm afraid.

Some areas seem bigger than they really are.

There is a self-involvement as in psychosis. I'm consumed with what I'm going through.

I felt better in the closet, I felt like myself again. It pulled me out of the state but it was also too compressed, it made the tremors start again in the upper shoulders.
O: Twitching and jerking of the shoulders.

A dull frontal headache, a digging in sensation.

A weird identity confusion. I looked in the mirror and didn't know who that was.

I don't like objects because they're too…like beings. They have too much energy being what they are. It's too impactful. I have a sensitivity as if my aura is expanding and all these objects are in my space.

O: Looking at a large shell
I feel like I could get really small and climb into the conch shell.

I like white and silver. I'm attracted to it. I can feel the energy vibrating from white.

Everything is too much. That seashell has too much power.
O: He backs away from it.

I feel the environment acutely, every geometry. It's like a funhouse. It's intriguing and disconcerting and panic making. Everything I look at is in a different light.
O: Looking up toward the ceiling and backing away.
It's like I know objects. I can speak to them. It's a feeling like a game. "Ha ha ha. Other people don't know you, lamp, but I know you." It's like a horror movie. Everything is alive. I feel like the existence of things is a little anthropomorphized. It's like a doll that's alive in horror movies - the picture, the lamp.

I'm acutely aware of a leaf moving across the driveway outside. It's hard to focus and remember well. When I replay things in my mind everything is a bit unstable.

It's like sitting in a subway station on white tile. Out of the darkness comes this blazing white light at great speed. Everything is fast and slippery. A feeling of speed. The whole house could shift. But there's also a dead, pallid, vacant, spooky feeling.

When I look at the ceiling it's like I'm much closer to it.

My way of relating to people would be to convey my bizarre relationship with objects. The relationship with objects is primary.

A dull headache, just sitting there like cement or rock, squeezing, worse on the right, better from pressing where the bones come together. It's from the middle of my head forward to above the eyebrows.
I love the colour white.

I don't like cobwebs. I like clean, minimalist, neo-modern angles and curves. The parsimony of it. I don't like clutter and dirt. I'm very interested in contour, lines, and design. I don't like mess. It's hectic, gross. I have an interest in interesting geometrics, there's something beautiful about it. I like arches. I could be an architect or interior designer. I like things sleek, crisp, and clean. I would love to be in a completely white room. Everything white. I want things sheer, sharp, and solid. I wouldn't want a rug. I think I would like glass, too; big skyscrapers stabbing the sky. There's something about white and dark.

I don't like to deal with people much. I have a real insecurity like I don't know how to do people, and a fear, but in another way I really don't care.

I might like a cat. Will you get the cat?

I could be haughty in an idiosyncratic way. There's a massive insecurity, but when I'm dealing with esthetics I'm in my milieu.

(speaking to the cat) We don't like people much, do we? Come here, precious. Come to daddy.

It would be interesting to have a cat but there's no strong draw. I'm more interested in the chair.

The remedy feels like it's poisonous, like it would deform blood cells. I have an image of the inside of a mouth. It's horrible, white ridges, puffy and inflamed.

I see others as rather pathetic? People are too complicated. They move, they have personalities and opinions. Why bother?

Irritation of the posterior nares.

There's a kid feeling; exploring the world and self-involved. A vulnerability because of not knowing how to deal with people. I feel like ordering, "do this", giving orders.

I feel inept socially but also superior. Both at the same time. I don't want to look at you. You're ludicrous. Most people are just garbage. They're clumsy, cluttered, and odorous. Like someone unshowered and sweaty. I have delicate white hands. An aristocrat looking at a peasant. It would be revolting but instead I just distance myself.

I like the word "pristine". I like things that rise.

(speaking with a very haughty, snobby tone)
Even though I'm loathe for some of these aspects, acutely aware of an immediate nature of all animate things which seem imperfect. The thing in itself as it were. Query me if you must.

There's a prudish quality. It's not like I want to rule the world. It's like Victorian discussions of how women should be white and pallid and refined. I'm very literary.

There's a fear of being the opposite of refined: gross, fat, white exudations, irregular skin, spots, moles. It's so incredibly gross to me. If I go into that mode I would never like myself. Never.

I have a feeling of being sickly and pallid. I might use a cane. I might not do well with changes of temperature, humidity, with weather in general. I'm an indoor creature.

The feeling as of a Victorian era aristocrat in England. Class, refinement, whiteness, purebred. Filth - you don't want it in your gene pool. Everything needs to be porcelain. There's no warmth toward other classes. I don't want to think about it. I don't want it in my presence.

I like Islamic art. The Taj Mahal. Geometric designs in white marble. I like pure geometry. I like it better than Greek sculpture.

A fascination for beautiful young boys, prepubescent. There's a beauty to their form before they get animal and hormonal. It's not necessarily to be sexual. It's more of a touch point. Perfection. Perfect proportions. They don't have the animal willfulness you get after puberty. The passivity and purity and harmony you have before that.

If I imagine myself as a women I have a hard time with sexuality. It's just animal and inherently dirty. A soft clean kiss on the lips is exquisite. But the thought of someone gyrating and coming inside me, ugh. I'm evaluating you all the time like a work of art. Are you good enough, your manners, knowing what's important to me, a good provider. I'm concerned about class. I'm like the Winona Ryder character in "The Age of Innocence".

Over time I can imagine one becomes very hard, like my facial expression. Dried up inside, rigid.

Irritation on the inside of the eyelids, where they touch the eyeballs.

So much about the remedy is about being alone. There's not much motive force, no engine. Except maybe for architecture or writing.

I can hear another voice. It's crass, loose, against refinement. It's a polarity, like trying to take a white straightjacket off. It wants mess, to take an axe to the windowsill, to paint the white lamp hippie colours, maybe a mural on the wall, wants a drooling dog, wants to sit in feces. A fascination with feces.

This has fright, not dread. This is cleaner and sharper. White fright. It's like fear in a crowd, on a bridge, in an enclosed space. Everything is unstable and moving quickly, it could move in or hurt you. It's not an assassin or a mugger, it's everything. The door or the window. The remedy is so bound up with objects and space. Everything could be right there, moving so quickly. It's a pure panic, the whole state is berserk. Just busy geometry is enough to create panic. Everything has this instability that could be panic making.

I want to be able to see 360 degrees around myself. There's a vulnerability about what I can't see. There's something about the upper back and neck; it's where I'm afraid of it getting me from behind.

Material things that suddenly hurt you. Objects become animate. They have no personality but they're not dead objects. They are alive and intriguing. They have form and substance. They're an entity.

I have a desire to chew the hell out of my nails, almost to rip them off.

I'm fretting. Rapid talk in my head.

Looking at the photograph of you on the wall - I don't want to look at it, there's too much going on, even the wood grain is too much.

Spinning (in swivel chair) ameliorates. Something automatic establishes stability and order. I can trick my senses. If I sit everything can shift and move. I'm at the whim of the shifting environment. With automatic motion all the flux is tempered, like if you're in a funhouse and it's freaking you out, and then you blur your eyes. The spinning is jamming the sensory input. There's something in particular about spinning. I want it to be very ordered.

If I don't like something I don't see why I should suffer through it. I don't want this, I want that. These things are loathsome, these are refined and give me pleasure. I want the loathsome to go away.

Pristine versus loathsome.

A feeling of "some things need measuring up here" (are in need of improvement). A desire for perfection. Not accumulating objects. There's an intolerance of second best.

If you went too far it's not refined, it's minimalist. Reducing, reducing, eliminating. I want all white paintings, but then I'm upset that there's a staple at the edge.

There was a French artist who only wrote 14 songs, they were masterpieces. Futzing until they're perfect. Then it looks garish so you reduce it further, trying to get rid of the gauche like a syphilitic washing his hands. If you stay with the finished product for too long it will start to look gauche and it has to be reduced again. Even a perfectly balanced asymmetry will need to be further refined because it's asymmetry.

An affinity for the sinus and oral membranes.
Painful earaches.
Joint pain like the bones are rubbing together.
A wheezing cough, slightly asthmatic.
A horrible taste in the back of the mouth, like a white rock or metal. It's like white gunk in the intestines, a little caustic. It's where the taste is coming from.

Intestinal blockage, irritation, discomfort, like white irritating gravel, irritating the tissue from the inside. The seat of action is in the intestines. The white stuff hangs out down there and causes trouble. It irritates the lining and disrupts metabolism.

Headache worse moving the head quickly.

I only want to spin to the right. To the left causes a headache.

The feeling about children would be - get a nanny.

With the aversion to loathsome things - oozing stuff is the worst.

I want a world where all the animals are white and dead and stuffed.

Prissy. Scandinavian architects. Fascination with light.

Tired and weak with joint complaints, like a person in an English novel who can't handle the weather, they're cold and susceptible.

An aversion to labor, and a feeling that it's beneath me, an aristocratic energy.

It reminds me of the practice of having sex through a hole in a sheet.

White light, purity, tall cathedrals full of glass and light.

How dare you incarnate me in an animal body. Insufferable the filth and disorder.

A love hate relationship with God - likes the absolute purity, but frustration that it hasn't been manifested.

There's something divine about a cat that becomes white in winter. It's so refined. It blanks out the animal markings and becomes pure. It's a metaphor for human transformation, what we are to be. There is such a beauty to that animal's form that it overcomes its animalness and becomes a work of art. I'm drawn to winter. The whiteness, snow, life is blanketed out, the crystalline snow structure, but not that I could tolerate it physically.

A snide, dissatisfied, invalid aristocrat with eccentric esthetics for purity.

Platina

Platina

Pride or Prejudice I

She tossed back her shiny blond hair to reveal beautifully formed features. Her tall body oozed sexuality, which was amplified by an attitude of command and disdain. The people at the party were in immediate awe of her authority; yet she displayed nothing but contempt towards them. "What am I doing here with these low-lifes?," she thought. "What a waste of precious time."

When we conjure up an image of Platina a certain personality comes to mind; a haughty sex goddess sneering contemptuously at puny mortals. Occasionally we may encounter a patient portraying this stereotypic image, but constricting our mind to a single concept will conceal many Platina cases. We can broaden this narrow perception by pinpointing the dynamic entity hidden at the centre of Platina's circle.

Our analysis begins at the split. Platina is one of the few remedies that has a delusion of being divided. This symptom should be differentiated from the delusion of being double. Division says 'my two sides', while double talks of 'two of me'. On a cellular level, doubling is the process of mitosis. Division occurs in sexual meiosis and results in two strands of DNA in search of partners.

Next we identify the dynamics generated around this split. The most consistent motion of Platina is alternation. This theme runs through the whole remedy:

joy	alternates	sadness
laughing	alternates	weeping
happiness	alternates	physical pain
sexuality	alternates	religion
physicals	alternate	mentals
melancholy	alternates	jesting
symptoms	alternate	sides

Rather then uniting both sides in a gentle and harmonious interchange, Platina alternates abruptly from one side to the other, a constant and rapid rotation across her division.
In the proving of Platina, the alternating moods are concomitant to the motion between a closed room and the open air. When outdoors she is cheerful and gay, but on entering the room she becomes melancholic, impatient, haughty and contemptuous.
This is accompanied by the typical delusion of being enlarged.

The polarity of inside and outdoors reflects the theme of constriction and enlargement in Platina. The narrow confines of the room constrict her soul, while the outside allows expansion into freedom and well-being. 'Out' and pleasure alternate with 'In' and displeasure. Her divided being is in a constant to and fro motion across the doorstep of joy and sadness, pleasure and pain, expansion and constriction. We can say that the doorstep represents the pivot of this Platina alternation. Other aspects of this 'doorstep' transition are fear of crossing the street and restlessness which drives her from place to place. An excellent image of the narrow tunnel between her two worlds is the typical 'hour glass contraction' of Platina's labour.

Rapid transition between extremes occurs when one aspect reaches maximum intensity and flips into its opposite. Just as ice burns at its coldest and fire becomes white at its hottest, extreme yang becomes yin and extreme yin flips into yang. In Platina's case, expansion expands to a point and constriction contracts into growth.

It is around this point of change that Platina alternates extremes. Dwelling near the precarious peak of the 6th period, she teeters from one side to the other. This affinity for change relates to platinum's characteristic as a chemical catalyst.

The larger Platina grows, the more she is constricted. She feels that she has been squeezed into a narrow space. Her pains are compressing, and she suffers from spasms, numbness and a sensation of being tightly bandaged. The characteristic fears of choking and hanging represent constricted air passages, along with a desire to whistle. The opposite polarity, expansion, is expressed by constant spasmodic yawning.

Platina, a dissected remedy, has an affinity with knives. Hahnemann states that this remedy should be prepared from 'chemically pure platina which is soft and can be cut with a knife.' If life were a knife, Platina would be the point. Ten thousand metallic molecules of blade compressed into an edge. Edge constricted to a tip, tip squeezed into a point. One single point; lonely, isolated, unique. The rest of the knife, handle, sheath and blade, all have one purpose - to serve the penetrating tip, without which a knife is useless. Do these lesser components appreciate this? Do they acknowledge her as the cutting edge? Do they perceive the singular role that only a purposeful piercing Platina point can play?

In the revolving wheel of life Platina's point of singularity lies at the reciprocal moments of birth and death. Many Platina symptoms revolve around labour, birth or post-partum. On the other hand we find symptoms of approaching death, death and murder. At times we find both together, as in 'Fear of killing during parturition' and 'Fear of death during delivery'.

Platina is aggravated around midnight, which is the time associated with these points of beginning and end, birth and death. The colour of midnight is black, which is the main discoloration produced by this remedy. Metallic platinum may be white or black.

During birth we are compressed through the smallest of corridors before expanding into the great outdoors. In the second stage of labour, transition, we are squeezed through the narrow os. This is the point of transition between the constricted room of pregnancy and the open spaces of life, love and light.

A similar process occurs during death. As life constricts our bodies shrivel, fruit withering to seed. Yearning for freedom from its confining shell, the soul is compressed out of the body. It squeezes through the narrow death canal, an os of tightly fused fontanelles, it emerging into the light of unrestricted love. Like a butterfly escaping its cocoon, it has transformed.

In order for life to evolve it must pass through narrow doorways. Old concepts are squeezed out as we compress through cramped openings. It is around these points of potential transformation that Platina alternates.

Death and birth are the narrow passages that enable us to let go of the old and move on to the new. These pivots of existence are represented by the sexual and crown chakras, which are the focus of Platina's pathology. Many personal and social transformations are initiated through the reciprocal power of sex and religion.

As Platina oscillates these catalytic cusps of change, sine waves cross horizontal axes, polarities reverse, antagonisms alternate, yin turns yang. Mannish girls laugh at serious matters, effeminate men enjoy sexual religion. Male exchanges female, symptoms extend crosswise, chills flush heat.

It is during this perpetual crossover that the pathological misplacement of Platina arises. Fearful for her beloved husband who has left the room, she imagines that he has had an accident and will never return. When he does, she feels estranged and would like to stab him. Returning after each transformative crossing she emerges into new and foreign places, away from home, a stranger in a strange land. From the proving: "She feels as if she did not at all belong to her family; after a short absence everything appears to be quite changed ...Imagines that she does not belong to this race."

Having left the room for a moment, she returns. But as she crosses the threshold it seems he is in new and strange surrounding. This is the wrong room! Like a foreigner in her own family or a tourist in the wrong country, left resides in right, yin has entered the house of yang.

There are points in our lives where unfamiliar new worlds catalyse a process of transformation. But has Platina really entered the wrong room? It seems much more likely that she has mutated during her absence, altering herself, but not her environment. A child who has been sent to boarding school returns, changed, to his old family. Nothing seems the same as it used to be. A teenager, touched by a spiritual experience, is alienated from her friends. A loving couple, separated for a while, rejoin as unfamiliar lovers. A soldier, back from the war, becomes the enemy of his own people. A child, fresh from other realms, imagines he is born to the wrong parents. A woman, emerging from puberty, realises she inhabits a man's body.

Platina's crossover into alien territory is evident on many levels. Demons invade her religious notions, while he desires anal coition with a woman. She dreams of strange places while familiar scenes seem horrible. Constipation away from home, prolapsed uterus, menses in old women.

Thus we find Platina, a stranger in a strange land, polarities reversed. Like Alice, she has stepped through the mirror and is living an inverted life. Alone in a bizarre world, estranged and isolated, she cries for help.

Pride or Prejudice II

She tossed back her shiny blond hair to reveal beautifully formed features. Her tall body oozed sexuality, amplified by an attitude of command and disdain. The people at the party were in immediate awe of her authority; yet she displayed nothing but contempt towards them. "What am I doing here with these low-lifes?" she thought.
"What a waste of my precious time."

The moment he appeared all that changed. He stood in the doorway, tall, elegant, imposing. His black clothes and hair matched her mood, and she felt his cold metallic gaze pierce her defences like a knife. Acutely aware of his radiant presence, she was overwhelmed by self-conscious embarrassment. She felt intensely oppressed by the crowded room, the irritating people, and her constricting dress. "What a man!" she thought, "He'll never talk to me, I'm just not in his league."

But he did. "Hi baby" he whispered, "How about a walk in the garden?" Though he phrased it as a question, she knew she had to obey. As soon as they stepped outside, she breathed a sigh of relief: "What a bunch of losers!"

A cigarette later and the conversation was becoming personal, with "sweetheart" "darling" and "beautiful". Her coolness soon melted under the warmth of his adoration.

"As soon as I saw you, I knew that you're the one for me, the only one. You are just so lovely." Suddenly he was down on one knee, "Be my princess, my goddess, let me worship you."

She felt irritated by this display of weakness. What a wimp! Why do people never live up to their image? She felt the old numbness creeping back into her heart. "P-leease! Don't be an idiot, get up. You're making a bit of a scene, aren't you?"

It was his turn to feel embarrassed. "Er... Sorry, I got a bit carried away." Why did no one appreciate his gallantry? He rose quickly, and though he towered above her, she knew she had him under control. "Get me a drink while I relax here in the open air." she commanded, lighting another cigarette. "Anything you say, princess", he said, and hurried back inside.

She strolled down the garden, whistling softly, proud of the way she had handled the situation. The sweet smell of irises lifted her spirit and expanded her mind.

Ten minutes later and he hadn't returned. "Jerk!" she murmured, walking back to the house. Entering the room through the narrow corridor she noticed that the atmosphere was different. The music and lights had changed, her friends had left and the remaining people seemed distant and unfamiliar. The air was stuffy, and she felt claustrophobic. Then she saw him, across the room, standing much too close to the beauty in the rainbow dress. "How dare he!" she thought, "Just who does he think he is!" She marched over…

"How could you! One minute you're sweet-talking me outside, and the next you're indoors whispering in some stranger's ear!"

He offered her a cursory glance, looking through her as if she didn't exist. "Do I know you?" and "Excuse us!" They turned away, and she thought she heard the rainbow queen snigger. Her mind felt numb. Again, rejected, again, humiliated. Again second best. Tears welled in her eyes as she rushed out.

But the cool air soon soothed her pain, and she began to see things from a different perspective. He really wasn't her type, a bit too plain. And he probably never would have accepted her operation anyway. Would people ever realise her true value?!

Alternative Platina

The original proving of Platinum, undertaken by Dr. Gross, appears in Hahnemanns' '*The Chronic Diseases*'. It is interesting to note that the majority of mental keynotes for which Platina is famous have been derived from a single prover, who has been described as "a very excitable young woman". Through generations of lesser materia medicas, the 'haughty woman' picture has been enlarged out of all proportion to other aspects of Platina. This narrow group of single prover symptoms has been confirmed in countless cases. From this we learn the importance and validity of a single prover's experience. Yet some modern homœopaths, who have had numerous successes based on this isolated prover, regard new provings which include such singular symptoms with contempt. If we were to follow their suggestions, cutting out all the unique experiences of individual provers, we would be left with a common proving of little value.

The following represent alternative points of view to the conventional Platina:

Past the Peak Platina

It is important to perceive that Platina's position is past the midpoint of the sixth period of the periodic table, and not actually at the peak. This lofty position is occupied by Iridium, the true queen of this realm. Iridium's stability comes from the certain knowledge that she is rightfully placed on the royal throne, a messenger between heaven and earth. Platina sits by her side, shiny and noble, but by no means monarch. Like her mother and grandmother, palladium and nickel, she is dressed for the part, but not internally validated. Subject to criticism and compliments, she needs constant appreciation to maintain her auxiliary position by the queen's side. Like any descendant of carbon, she is essential to those around her, but painfully dependent upon their recognition.*

Thus the Platina loftiness is opposed by a sense of embarrassment, disgrace and humiliation, internal feelings of those who look the part but are not it. Like noblemen at the king's side, they aspire to his position, but are shamefully constricted by the knowledge that it is not theirs by birthright. Platina is prone to suffer from deceived ambition, self reproach, neglected feelings and a delusion that she is unworthy to live.

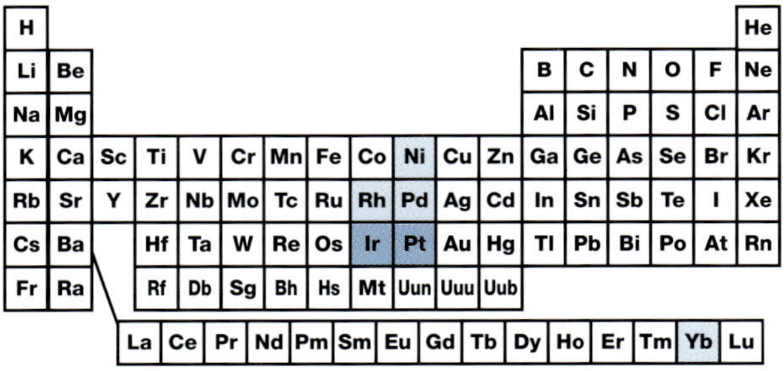

* The conflict of leadership (mid-period, according to Scholten) between Iridium and Platina is complicated by the fact that the mid-point calculation of the period often considers the lanthanides (elements 57 – 71) as one element. If we include the lanthanides, ytterbium (element 70) would be in the centre. It is easier to calculate according to the period above. If we count without the noble xenon, then rhodium, iridium's mother, is situated in the center of the period. However, when including the noble gas, the middle of the fifth period is actually between rhodium and palladium. If we consider the noble gas as the jester, we can say that the presence of the jester devalues the king and elevates the nobles.

Proceedings of the American Institute of Homœopathy, "Platina," by Dr. V. Meyer.

Whether Platina is suitable only for irritable, excitable females, with predominant activity of the sexual functions, as the majority of writers assume, and among them Stapf and Gross, the provers of it, who, by the way, made their provings on a very excitable young woman, I shall leave undetermined. For myself, I have had frequent occasion to administer Platina, and have obtained the very best curative results in appropriate diseased conditions, occurring in phlegmatic women of lax fibre. This observation, too, appears to me to stand by no means in opposition to the totality of the Platina symptoms, but rather to accord most clearly with them. For, on a critical review of what has been made known concerning the action of the remedy, we find that all of by far the greater part of its symptoms bear the character of depression, but not that of erethism. A lack of energy, a lack of electric tension of the nerves, if I may so express myself, seem to me more clearly manifest in Platina than in any other remedy. And although we find, it is true, isolated phenomena which seem to indicate a contrary action, yet we regard these only as reflex or alternate effects; and, indeed, they occur in so isolated a manner as almost to disappear before the mass of symptoms which justify the view I have taken.

It may be that a farther proving of this drug, which, by the way, is very desirable *(my emphasis – JS)*, would disprove our assumption: for the present, however, we can only hold to that proving of which we are already in possession. In this proving, we find, in every system on which Platina acts, the stamp of relaxation, of diminished energy, of depression, of torpor. As well in the psychical and sensuous, as in the sensitive, motor and vegetative nervous systems, we see this character manifested by the trembling, the sensations of chilliness, the coldness and paralysis which are so frequently present.

Extracts from the Proving of Platinum 1980

Dr O.A. Julian's proving of Platinum has been based on the Hahnemannian method, using his own established experimental protocol, further details of which may be found in *Homeopathie – Collection Abreges* by O.A. Julian and M. Haffen (ed. Masson, 1981).

The number of provers was 55, 21 women and 34 men. The trial was done blind, using random allocation. In addition, 5 subjects received placebo only. The potencies used were 30CH, 7CH, 4CH, and placebo.

(*Italics* – O.A. Julian, **bold** type – J. Sherr)

Fatigue: *periodic*, when getting up in the morning; a permanent ***desire*** **to sleep**; the *whole body* feels **drowsy** after an effort of *sustained concentration*; at the end of the afternoon with *burning* sensations which radiate towards the shoulders and the head; *general*, **lacks drive** for working, and the shoulders, back of neck, back and arm muscles feel painfully *heavy*; washing is an effort, feels like *crying*; is completely *indifferent* as regards watching T.V.

Physical or intellectual work is *depressing* in the morning; **fatigue** *worse* in the evening between 8p.m. and 11p.m.; when *talking*; by prolonged conversation with constant necessity to **yawn**; caused by a slight effort even to speak.

Needs to *smoke*; *aches* and *pains* generalized; it's difficult to get up in the morning; *criticizes* more than usual; feels that the *heart is about to "pack up"*; feels *sick* and *discomfort* all over after massage of a painful shoulder; feels *unwell* when travelling by car; uncontrolled *desire* for *sweet* dishes; the *head* is "*fuddled*", the shoulders feel heavy, *perspiration*.

Hesitation, indecision, pains all over and feels like *weeping*.
All activity, physical or mental, is *repugnant* about 10 a.m.
Works but has not drive, works "without pleasure".
Is bad-tempered, no taste for reading; *doesn't wish to watch thrillers* on T.V.
Is often *irritable*, has difficulty in concentrating.
Is in **poor spirits**, "**down in the dumps**", feels like crying.
Sadness: looks as though he is *sad*; feels sad; lacks joy, *fed up with living and fed up with all that makes life; nothing interests him*; is sad, ***weary to death***; feeling of **boredom**, "*spleen*".
Depression: is *depressed*, feels awful; *looks on the* ***black*** *side of things,* is disturbed by his environment; tends to be depressed and has suicidal thoughts; becomes more and more ***bored***, **wishes to** ***die***.

Feeling of frustration: **empty** feeling, lacks something in the stomach; feels *better* when "**too full**" but is *worse* after, because smitten with **remorse at not having resisted the impulsion to eat.**
Everything goes against him, is often **bored.**
Feels out of sorts in the *morning*, irritated, everything goes wrong, has a throbbing feeling in the arteries.
Continues to feel out of sorts in the afternoon and the throbbing feeling in arms and legs continues also.
Nothing goes right, **nothing interests him**, wishes to die and *thinks* that he would be *happy if he saw his death about to happen.*

Degradation of self; urge to **destroy oneself and others**; a recurring obsessed state; is not clear-headed and has fixed ideas. Feels that the environment and the **family circle** *are deteriorating*. Criticizes, is *lucid* about himself and his **circle**; his *family circle* appears "*illogical*", becomes *unfamiliar* to him; *feels different* compared to other people, especially as regards the family. Feels *lucid* compared to other people; the **family circle is "unfamiliar"**. Feels "*disconnected*" *from himself and other people.* Constantly feels as though he is in a trance.

Becomes more *aggressive*, tendency to say aloud what he thinks about someone or something. Observes himself becoming *nasty*. Is in low spirits *contradictory*; wants to be alone and then wishes for company. *Everything goes* ***wrong***, **joyless**, **bored**, **wishes to die.** ***Shuts himself up*** in his room to avoid conflicts. *Doesn't wish to do anything,* ***doesn't feel at home anywhere***, not even in his home. Prefers to remain alone in his room. *Very weary*, unable to cope with the daily housework so the house becomes very untidy and disorderly. *Violent conflicts* with the family who reproach her for laziness; this attitude *exasperates* her and increases her **desire to die**. Is *bad-tempered*, irritated by visitors; neglects toilet and clothes. Is *"absent", not present. Fierce, aggressive,* talks aloud to himself when walking.
Is *annoyed* by arguments with his **family circle**.
Apprehensive, has no will-power; *undecided*, unable to carry out his work. *Apathetic*, lacks coordination, refuses all contacts with his family. *Dissatisfied.* Constantly *worried*, anxious.

Disorders in the perception of time: thinks that he is early and then finds out that he is just on time. ***Has the feeling of living "outside" time.*** Has the *impression* that he is ***destroying himself***, sees himself becoming *nasty*. Generalized discomfort in the body, particularly on the right side, feels ***bored*** the whole time. *Half conscious state, has absences* and his *recollections are vague.*

Tendency to put on weight, *with* **bulimia**.

Face and *eyelids* are ***swollen***, the internal part of eyelids also.
The *lower eyelids* are so **swollen** that they cover the lower edge of the spectacles.
Aches and pains all over, fatigue, *suffocation*, **puts on weight** (1 kg in one night).
Doesn't feel hungry, but his "brain wants to eat".
Uncontrolled urge **to eat so as to feel "full".**
As he becomes fatter, feels more and more awful.
Face is ***bloated****, hands* ***swollen*** and painful.
Weight increased by 6 kg during the 4 weeks of the proving.
Drowsiness in the daytime.
Voraciously hungry about 5 p.m., satiated by eating **1 kg of ice-cream**.
Cellulitis on internal side of upper part of thighs, **double chin, size of waist increases, big stomach.** ***Empty feeling*** **in the** ***stomach*** one hour after dining.
Strong urge for **sweet dishes**.
Face is swollen, creased with many wrinkles.
Hands swollen, particularly the right one.
Weight varies, loses and then **puts on weight** but normal (good) diuresis is maintained.
All his ***clothes*** **seem** ***tight***.
Pulse is quickened.
It feels as though a needle has been driven into the right side of his Adam's apple. **He** ***feels as though he has left (been outside) his body*** **during the night**. Having made an effort to concentrate, he has the impression that a "*ball*" is *going upwards towards his head and is going inside his skull,* ***swelling*** *up* at the same time.

Sleep: Disturbed: insomnia – he cannot stop thinking about past events in his life. Insomnia because of *fixed ideas*; sleep is agitated, with nausea. *Wakes up in the middle of the night* with a feeling of ***fatigue*** **and aching** all over. *Takes a long time* getting off to sleep. Is *half-asleep* with wandering thoughts. Wakes up about 3 a.m. feeling very thirsty. *Wakes up in the middle of the night* with the feeling that he "***has left his body***". This feeling continues and recurs. *Is either* long or quick getting off to sleep. *Is half asleep, hears* people moving around him and has to *make a big effort to open his eyes*. After a prolonged sleep he feels *dazed*. Sleep is agitated, *difficult* to get off to sleep, unable to find a suitable position. Sleep is very agitated, *wakes up a lot*, needs to urinate, the stomach has a **heavy feeling** and moving about is difficult. ***Insomnia*** **and feel bored, has an urge to eat**, and has polyarticular pains. *Wakes up early* about 6.30 a.m., because he is cold, needs to urinate and has a stomach ache.
Bilateral sciatica or *unilateral right*, worse at night.
Lacks assurance. Is ***unable to calculate and estimate distances easily.*** **Is unable to drive a car.** *Trembles* all over and has to rest in bed.
Feels his heart beating, particularly when reading, and has the ***feeling*** **that** ***he is outside his body.***

Analogy: The Cuckoo

The common cuckoo of Europe and Asia, Cuculus canorus, is the species whose two-note call has been invoked in many musical compositions as well as in cuckoo clocks. This species, like many other cuckoos, is a brood parasite; the female lays her eggs in the nests of smaller birds who raise the young cuckoos, usually at the expense of the rightful occupants of the nest.

Young cuckoos reach maturity only with the help of foster parents. When an adult female is ready to lay her eggs, she looks among the nests of other birds in her territory until she finds one with new eggs of a similar shape, size, and colour to her own. While the resident birds are away from the nest, she then removes an egg and lays one in its place, carrying the stolen egg away for a meal. The stowaway cuckoo almost always develops and hatches before its foster brothers and sisters. It uses this advantage to get rid of its competition, either by ejecting all other objects (eggs or chicks) from the nest or by trampling the others once they have hatched. The Cukoo's beak, which is much larger than the host species, deceives the parents into thinking they are feeding many mouths. These amazing characteristics ensure that the foster parents focus all of their reproductive energy on the cuckoo.

Cuckoo clocks utilise a mechanical cuckoo that ejects through a narrow door every hour. Some have male and female figures which alternate.

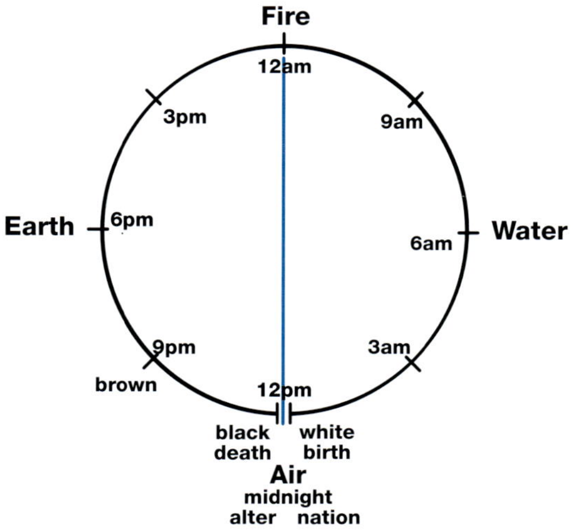

Platina Synthesis

Julian's Proving

Verb

Sensation:
Outside the circle: Body, family, time. Cannot enter or connect.
Emptiness inside the circle. Tedium.

Function:
Must enter the circle. Must fill himself. Enlargement, swelling, bulimia.

Hahnemann's Proving (Dr. Gross) and Julian's Proving

Verb

Sensation:
In strange surroundings.

Function:
Must exit – Must enter.

Noun

Doorway, threshold. Knife.

Related Rubrics

Mind; dreams; acquaintances, distant
Mind; dreams; acquaintances, distant; strange things
Mind; dreams; country; foreign
Mind; dreams; unsuccessful efforts to; reach a distant place
Mind; emptiness of the mind, sensation of
Head; falling of head; out, sensation as if contents would be falling out of head
Mind; unconsciousness, coma; general; emptiness, with feeling of
Stomach; emptiness, goneness, hungry feeling
Chest; empty sensation
Generalities; emptiness, hollow sensation
Chest; fullness; general; stuffed, as if
Stomach; fullness
Generalities; full feeling; internal

Stillingia Sylvatica

Image:
Sylvatica Syphilitica

A fantasy for Stillingia

Still, the night bends,
silver moon
sends,
a sliver,
darting, shimmering,
spidery shadowlight
dances its beam.
Sylvatica, delighted,
crowns her queen
lady syphilis,
(with)
laurels
of sterling moonbeam.

Still night,
stiletto,
shining silver,
darts, stabs,
touches bone,
penetrates.
The queen
is dead,
silver crown rolling to the ground.

All hail syphilis,
King of dark.

Stillingia Sylvatia

The finest and most accurate way to study remedies is reading provings, **the root** of all true materia medica. **Burning** desire **fertilises** our intellect and imagination, **nourishing** the **delights** of perception. However, studying provings may appear daunting due to the overwhelming amount of information, especially if the proving has few striking or mental symptoms. Thus many homœopaths forgo the **deeper** understanding of provings and opt for superficial remedy pictures.

As in case taking, the study of provings is an art. We **sharpen** our minds, **penetrating** through long sentences to essential ideas and expressions. Surfing the bland language of symptoms, we follow individual ideas **down towards** collective **roots**, searching for common denominators. We remain conscious of characteristic words and expressions that **dart** and **protrude** through the surface like **nodes**, seeking our attention.

These expressions are often those that might seem unimportant to the non-homœopathic reader. Rather than focusing on gross pathology, common emotions, subjects and nouns, we unfocus our gaze on verbs, idioms and analogies, so as to perceive more subtle aspects. In this way, the student of materia medica can study long and tedious provings without attempting to memorise all the symptoms.

I have used Stillingia to illustrate this concept, as it is a little known and underproved remedy. Surprisingly, it is a **black type syphilitic** remedy. This is even more unusual for a **plant**, as most intensely **syphilitic** remedies are **metals**.

A well proved remedy will emphasise its own characteristics, but our materia medica contains many bland provings. The exercise of this chapter is to demonstrate the difference between reading the tedious totality of a proving and distilling its essential features, including sensation and function. Using the introduction and abbreviated proving from, Clarke's *Dictionary* and extracts from the original proving, I have highlighted the symptoms that characterise this remedy for me. The poems are loose impressions that **stem** from the **underlying** facts.

Stillingia Sylvatica

Extracts from Clarke's *Materia Medica*

(all emphasis mine – JS)

Stillingia sylvatica, Linn.
Natural order: **Euphorbiaceae**.
The tincture is prepared from the **root** of the **Queen's Delight**, a perennial plant found in Virginia, Florida and a few other neighboring states.

Still. has long been a popular remedy for **syphilis** in the southern states of U. S.
The proving was from chewing the **root** or taking the tincture.

The proving shows an action closely **parallel** with that of **syphilis**, attacking the genito-urinary organs, throat (pharynx, larynx, and trachea), mouth, head, and bones.
I have cured with it **syphilitic** cough of the hoarse, barking type.
Still. attacks the **periosteum** and produces pain in the bone.
It has removed nodes on the forehead, **tibia**, and elsewhere, and arrested **caries** of the **nasal bones**.
Pain in the **cranial bones** and the headaches of **syphilis**.

It has a popular repute in scrofula, skin affections, liver diseases, and rheumatism – all of which the provings confirm.

In chronic rheumatism Hale classes it with **Phyt. and K. iod.**
Peculiar sensations are: As of a **heavy substance** pressing on brain.
Tongue as if **scalded**.
As if room were too warm.
Pains are **sharp**, **shooting**, **darting**.

Hale quotes a case of **secondary syphilis** treated by Preston, one of the provers.
The patient, a man, suffered extreme **torture** from **bone pains**. After receiving Still. he **slept** well.

The immense **nodes** disappeared from head and legs, and "from the most **deplorable, down-hearted** (sometimes almost raving from derangement), **miserable, thin-looking object**, he changed into a buoyant, joking, rotund-looking fellow." **The symptoms were worse by movement**.

Clinical

Bones, diseases of, nodes on.
Clergyman's sore throat.
Elephantiasis.
Hemorrhoids.
Headaches, syphilitic, mercurial, catarrhal.
Hip-joint disease.
Influenza.
Larynx, affections of.
Liver, affections of.
Nodes.
Periostitis.
Psoriasis.
Rheumatism.
Scrofula.
Syphilis.

Mind

Depression of spirits, and gloomy forebodings.
Intellect dull and stupid.

Head

Dizziness and throbbing in head.
Persistent dull headache in vertex.
Dull, heavy pain in right side of head.
In frontal region a feeling as of a heavy substance pressing on brain, becoming sharp and darting, almost unendurable.
Pains in head, with inflamed and watery eyes, and **general soreness of muscles.**
Sharp darting pains in right occipital protuberance.
Mercurial, syphilitic, and catarrhal headaches.
Bone swellings in head and forehead, in latter size of hen's eggs.
Mercurial periostitis of skull.

Eyes

Eyes inflamed and watery, with severe headache and general muscular soreness, as if he had taken cold.
Sharp darting pain over left eye, lachrymation of both eyes, especially after reading, right eye aggravates.

Ears

Burning in left ear in evening, next morning a vesicular eruption.

Nose

Catarrhal discharge, first watery then muco-purulent, followed by small abscesses on inside of right nostril.
Sharp burning sensation in right nostril, 6 A.M. on waking.
Influenza.
Necrosis of bones of nose.

Face

Pains under **malar bone**, extending **transversely** through face. **Stinging darting pains in face**, with frontal headache.
Periostitis of facial bones.

Mouth

Paroxysms of **neuralgic toothache.**
Scalded sensation on tongue, with soreness in region of larynx.
Heat in mouth and fauces.
Increased flow of saliva.

Throat

Smarting, stinging, dryness and rawness of fauces.
Constriction of throat.
Intense burning in fauces and throat extending to stomach, worse on any attempt to swallow.

Stomach

Appetite: increased, lost.
Regurgitation and vomiting of ingesta.
Pyrosis daily, 3 p.m. to bedtime.
Nausea with constipation.
Sickness and salivation.
Faint, **empty sensation in stomach.**
Distress, griping, cramps in stomach.

Abdomen

Torpidity of liver with jaundice, great depression, constipation.
Severe cramps in both hypochondria.
Sharp darting in left hypochondrium, followed by passage of flatus.
Borborygmi.
Colic, periodical.
Heavy pain in hypogastric region.

Stool

Pain in rectum and sphincter with stool, **burning and tenesmus.**
Bowels loose and irregular.
Stools: copious, acid, frothy, bilious, papescent, white like curds, dysenteric.
Constipation, stools delayed.

Urinary

Dull **pain in region of kidneys**.
Incontinence of urine.
Violent **smarting burning through whole length of urethra** worse by micturition, with difficulty in voiding urine.
Urine: increased, flocculent, mucous sediment.

Male genitalia

On micturating, **sharp pain in glans extending up urethra, so severe as to cause perspiration.**
Slight drawing up in right testis.
Dull tearing pain in left testis.
Gonorrhoea.

Female genitalia

Both ovaries pained very severely.
Copious muco-purulent leucorrhoea, with rheumatic pains.

Respiration

Laryngitis, especially if syphilitic, with hoarseness and dry spasmodic cough, or cough may be loose.
Hoarseness and chronic laryngeal affections in public speakers.
Croup.
Slight uneasiness and tickling in trachea and bronchi, worse on rising in morning.
Tickling sensation in trachea in evening which causes dry, spasmodic cough.
Slight lame feeling seemingly in cartilages of larynx.
Hoarse cough.
Bruised feeling in trachea.
Short, hacking cough.
Cough deep and loose.

Chest

Oppression of chest.
Darting pain in thorax, with tickling in throat and short, hacking cough.
Sharp darting pains through chest and shoulders.
Sore aching above left clavicle.
Raw feeling in chest whole length of sternum.
Incipient phthisis in persons of strumous habit.

Heart

Boring pains about region of **heart**, with irregular pulse.
Pulse weak and very irregular.

Back

Aching in back and **down thighs and legs**.
While sitting pain in left lumbar region, **darting forwards**.

Upper limbs

Sharp **shooting** pains in both arms, from middle third of humerus down to fingers.
Very large node on **olecranon**.
Aggravating pains in left elbow, shooting towards shoulder and head, slighter in right elbow and wrist.

Lower limbs

Aching pain in right leg.
Pains in left lower anterior third of leg.
Burning-itching of legs.

Enlargement of tibia to such a degree as to **deprive the child of all power of motion, limbs contracted and swollen.**
Ulcers on legs, venereal, chronic, and indolent.
Periostitis and nodes of tibia.
Syphilitic and gonorrhoeal sciatica, left sided complaints.
Legs and feet feel tired, and feet sore.

Sleep
Unusual drowsiness all day, with general malaise and headache.
Very sleepy after eating.

Fever
Cold on going to bed, immediately after broke out in sweat, with excessive warmth all night.
Feverish heat, evening.
Fever 1 A.M., gets into heavy sleep.
During day, room felt too warm.
Great warmth in face like catarrhal fever.

Skin
Itching and burning-itching of legs worse exposure to air.
Vesicular eruption on ears.
Scrofulous, venereal, and other skin diseases.
Ulcers with unhealthy skin.
Elephantiasis.
Lepra.

Relationships
Antidote to: **Merc.**
Antidoted by: **Ipec.** (nausea from the fumes).
Compare: In **syphilis, Syph., Med., Merc., K. iod.**
Chronic rheumatism, **Guaiac., Phyt.** Nodes, Mang., Corydalis, Staph. Hip disease, Nat. s.

EXTRACTS FROM ALLEN'S *ENCYCLOPEDIA*

General and Mind

Soreness of the muscles all over; feels as if he had taken a severe cold.
Feel quite distressed. **Felt miserable** all the forenoon.
Felt weak and emaciated, as if I had lost all my strength and energy.
Feel very languid, having great desire to sleep; Dull heavy feeling all over, especially in both legs; feel sore from the top of my head to the soles of my feet; don't want to move; want to go where I will not be annoyed; the duties of my profession are irksome; head feels heavy; perfect relaxation of all the muscles of the neck; my brain feels too large for the skull; requires considerable exertion to keep my eyes open.
Suffered from a general feeling of **malaise** about bedtime, but somewhat improved upon waking, after sleeping all night. **Depression of spirits** and **gloomy forebodings. Low spirits.**
Intellect dull and stupid.

Head

A feeling as if a **heavy substance was pressing** on the brain, the front part; the pain became very **sharp and darting**, in fact, almost unendurable.
Violent frontal headache.
Slight frontal headache.
Headache, in the evening; a constant **flowing pain**, like a **current, running** from the **median line** of the forehead to the **occipital process** and left cerebellum; this symptom was noticed several days since.
Severe sharp shooting in right side of frontal bone, **running downward** to the eye.
Sharp darting pain in the sinciput, extending to the occiput
Slight headache, **running** from anterior portion of temples; the pain is dull and constant.
A slight, constant, dull pain through the temples and forehead.
Darting pain in the left temporal region, **as if a piece of wire or some sharp-pointed instrument had been thrust into the temples.**
Sharp darting pain in the right occipital **protuberance**.

Eyes

Sharp darting pain over the left eye, with slight lachrymation from both eyes, more profuse when reading; right eye affected more than left.

Nose

Woke at 6 A.M. feeling a s**harp burning sensation** in the right nostril.

Face

Pain under malar bone, extending **transversely** through the face.
Stinging-darting pains in the face.

Mouth and Teeth

Spells of **neuralgic toothache.**
Considerable heat in mouth and fauces, extending **down** the oesophagus, with burning in the stomach.
Salty taste in the mouth.
Bitter taste in the mouth, in the morning.
The taste of this **root** is **pungent**, and leaves on the **root of the tongue** and fauces an impression **biting and irritating**, exciting a flow of **saliva.**
Increased flow of saliva.

Throat

Smarting and stinging in the fauces, after an hour subsiding, leaving a feeling of **rawness and smarting** in them; dryness of the fauces; smarting, stinging, and dryness of the fauces all day.
Intense **burning** feeling in the fauces and throat, which extended to the stomach; felt as if the whole surface had been **deprived of its epithelium**, causing an **intense burning** sensation when any attempt to swallow was made; this sensation continued in the stomach two hours; slight burning sensation in the stomach.
Slight warmth of the fauces.
Considerable heat in the fauces, which gradually increased until the throat became very sore.

Stomach

Pyrosis coming on each day about **3 P.M.** and lasting until bedtime.
Pyrosis was a constant attendant while proving the remedy, commencing about **2 P.M.** and continued until bedtime.
Nausea and vomiting.

If we remain in a closed room where the root is being boiled, and the vapor passes into the room, a sense of sickness at the stomach is excited, with a disposition to discharge saliva, with headache and other unpleasant symptoms.

Sick and qualmish at the stomach; sickness relieved by Ipecac.

Abdomen

Sharp darting pain in the left hypochondrium; appears to **begin in the ascending colon and passes through the transverse into the descending colon**, followed by escape of flatus.
Colic like pains; violent pains in the umbilical region.
Constant rumbling in the bowels, **relieved by escape of flatus.**
Sharp darting pains in my bowels.

Rectum

For several days after taking the last dose, **had severe attack of piles**, the first I had ever suffered.
Pain in the **sphincter ani**, as though the muscle had been bruised.
On voiding stool, very severe **burning at the anus and considerable tenesmus.**
With the loose evacuations, great **tenesmus and burning at the anus.**

Stool

Diarrhoea.
After a short time my **bowels became very loose** and irregular; this condition was soon followed by constipation, accompanied with nausea, together with a slow and irregular pulse when lying down; subsequently, a sensation as though diarrhoea were about to set in.
Two copious, acrid, frothy, bilious evacuations from by bowels, with some **tenderness and a burning sensation** in the anus; at **2 P.M.**
A diarrhoeic stool followed by griping pains in the epigastrium.

Urinary

On waking at 6 A.M., **sharp darting pain in both kidneys,** the left first, and then the right, with dull heavy pain in the left testicle.
Severe pain in the right kidney, or in its immediate vicinity, the pain, however, of short duration.
Violent smarting-burning pains throughout the entire length of the urethra, aggravated by micturition, with difficulty in voiding urine, and dull **pain in region of kidneys**; the pains continued for two hours so severe that it was **impossible to remain quiet.** Pain in the urethra severe at times and during micturition; can detect no discharge.

Male

Sharp pains in the penis on waking.
Slight **drawing up** of the right testicle.
Dull heavy pain in the left testicle.

Heart

Boring pains about the region of the heart.

Back

Aching pains in back, **extending down** the **thighs and legs**, in the evening.
While sitting, some pain in left lumbar region, **shooting from behind forward.**

Extremities

Suffering from great soreness of bones and muscles of extremities, caused by severe exercise; the soreness was greatly increased, and great aching of the extremities was experienced.
Pain in the right shoulder blade, **running up** the neck.
Sharp shooting pains in both arms, from **middle third of humerus down to fingers.**
Aggravating pains in **left elbow, extending towards shoulder and hand**, as though the bones were sore and would separate; slighter pains, of like character, in right elbow; aching also in left **carpal and metacarpal bones**; these pains are temporarily relieved by change of position.
Sharp pains in bend of left elbow, increased by **hanging down**.
Pain in right elbow, forearm, and wrist, **aggravated by motion**.
Sharp shooting pains in upper third and inner side of forearm, aggravated by letting **limb hang down**, and relieved by pressure, at 9.30 A.M.
Aching pain on outside of right thigh and leg, **running down to foot.**
Stabbing in right knee.
Drawing pain in the left knee, affecting the gastrocnemius.
Sharp darting pain in the right ankle-joint, outer part.
Pain in **both external malleoli**.
Severe pains in right foot, increased on standing and **attempting to walk**, in upper part of foot over the instep.
While in the house, pain in the **third toe** of the right foot.
While walking, pain in metatarsal joint of great toe, **running back to heel**, in both feet.

Skin

The juice of the **root** applied to the **surface** and rubbed upon it, occasions **smarting** and **irritation.**
The first symptom experienced which I thought might be attributable to the action of the drug, was a **burning itching of the legs**, below the knees, which seemed much worse by exposure to the atmosphere.

Roots

Deep
beneath the ground,
searching,
extracting nourishment,
where others dare not go.
Pushing, grinding, mining,
I penetrate
treacherous grounds,
determined, unacknowledged,
I bore on.

Never summoning
nor expecting
enlightened ray of cowardly light
to follow,
I twist and curl,
groping my way
through convoluted terrain.
Home
is my living grave.

Yet even as I grasp the hand of Hades
hardening my heart
like metal,
against the pain,
eternal night.
I know
that all, yes all, above me,
thrives, survives,
by me.

I am the root.

And what of bone
my brother,
lying deep below the surface,
lending structure, feeding,
sucking on our mother's marrow
hiding face in shame.
An ulcer may penetrate,
bearing shafts of light,
that will illume
our secret hidden deeds;
destruction.
We rip and tear,
consume,
and gorge our way through rubble,
so that you
in pretentious innocence,
may grow.

From Fracastoro's 'Syphilis'

"Ilceus, my darling, who in the extremity of your sufferings have at least been heard by the Gods, you can hope for no salvation wherever the Sun gazes over the wide earth. This is the form of punishment Diana, Goddess of the Crossroads, metes out to you, and Apollo, won over by the prayers of Diana, on account of the sacred stag struck by a javelin near our stream, whose bristling head you fixed to our tree's stem. For after she saw the wild creature sprawled lifeless on the grass with its head cut off, and the fields sprinkled with its sacred blood, she made lament in all her woods and uttered dreadful curses against the author of the crime. Leto's son attended to his sister's grim prayers and both unrelenting sent this abominable plague upon you to make you wretched; furthermore they also refused you help anywhere the sun gazes; so if any salvation exists it must be sought in the depths of the earth below, beneath night's darkness.

... Then he prayed to Night and the Goddesses of Night, powers unknown.

... Ilceus (for neither your name nor your shameful illness is unknown to me not the reason for your coming), divest your heart of fear, our dear beloved Callirhow does not send you here in vain; salvation has been devised for you in the earth's depths. Lift up your spirits and follow me through the dark silences of the earth;

... All of this which opens up before you is Earth in all its vastness: the whole of the lightless world, realms in thrall to night, gods inhabit; the lowest habitations are kept by Proserpine, the highest by rivers which roused from their sacred caves pass echoing through the wide earth to the sea. In the middle are the rich Nymphs from whom are born the families of metals, the source of copper and silver and gleaming gold. I myself, who came to you in pity, am one of these sisters,..."

'Neighbours, it was with a knife,
just a little knife,
that on the appointed day between two and three,
two men in love killed each other.
With a knife,
just a little knife,
that fits snug in the hand
and slices so quickly
through the startled flesh
to stop at the point
where the dark root of the scream
lies trembling enmeshed.'

Federico Garcia Lorca, '*Blood Wedding*'

Stillingia Synthesis

Verb

Sensation:
Running, flowing, up and down.

Function:
Must be still, can not walk, can not move.

Sensation:
Heavy and enlarged, pressing.

Function:
Must contract, sharp, shoot, dart.

Form

Triangle: tibia, nose, node, elbow, olecranon, malleoli.
'Sharp pointed instrument'.
Triangle represents forward motion (tibia, nose).

Noun

Root, bone.

Syphilinum

Syphilinum Analysis

Nosode

Dr. Feller said it was absurd to claim that any disease could be cured by its nosode. …The only way, therefore, to use a nosode is to prove it on the healthy, like any other drug, and note its symptoms in the regular way.

Lines

- Headache: linear, from or near one eye backward; lateral; frontal; from temple to temple; deep into brain from vertex; as from pressure on vertex.
- Headache through temples, thence vertically like an inverted letter T.

Parallel Lines

- Constant linear headache, commencing at both angles of forehead and extending in parallel lines backward - a precursor of epileptic attack.
- Pain from eyes through to occiput.
- Diplopia, one image seen below the other.
- Tongue red and thick; two deep cracks running lengthwise in it; one on each side of median line.
- Two large ulcers, one on each side near apex of tongue.
- Two indurated ulcers at mouth of anus somewhat sore.
- Pain as if in kidneys, seemingly traversing ureters, but instead of passing into bladder followed spermatic cord, down groins and into testes.
- Two abscesses in groin.
- Two ulcers larger than a crown piece, dirty stinking, sloughing, with jagged, elevated edges are on thigh above patella, another on head of tibia; two large pieces of bone came away from head of tibia.
- After retiring, nerve chill beginning in anus, running down legs with spasmodic sensation.
- Skin; eruptions; symmetric (C)
- Generalities; symmetrical complaints (C)
- Arithmetical calculations difficult. X+Y=Z.

Syphilinum

Syphilinum is one of the remedy portraits that have strayed far from their source. When pure provings are deficient or insufficiently studied, clinical information and idle theories take on lives of their own. Rather than growing organically from original data, hypotheses develop in parallel to it. To move safely forward, we would do well to re-study the proving, developing diverse ideas upon a single solid base.

The popular 'essence' of Syphilinum is of ritualistic and obsessive behaviour, fear of bacteria and aversion to dirt, as well as guilt, violence and propensity to accidents – is this image fact or fiction? None of this information appears in the original proving. At best, these additions have been derived from accurate clinical observation and thoroughly cured symptoms. At worst, they are constructed from flights of fancy, fuelled by the need to fill gaping holes in our materia medica. building our house on rock rather than sand.

Syphilinum is generally prescribed on well known keynotes: Obsessive hand-washing, despair of recovery, alcoholism, nightly aggravations and bone pains. But what is the pattern that unites this apparently diverse information? How do these many parallel features coverge into one theme? It is common these days to search for an underlying psychological factor. However, if we can find a simple blueprint, a line of logic spanning both physical and mental symptoms, we may be able to discover the single point from which the whole remedy emanates.

What force weaves together fear of insanity, inaptitude for mathematics, despair of recovery? What idea unites aggravation from storms, amelioration in the mountains, serrated and pointed teeth? What is the common denominator combining affections of the middle finger, convergent strabismus, pains at insertion of deltoid? What connects the diverse symptoms of washing the hands, ovarian pains at the point of orgasm, symmetrical eruptions? What are the parallels concealed within the symptoms? Rather than founding our hypothesis on elusive mentals, let us head down the physical trail in search of a clue.

The Syphilinum headaches are worse at night, as are the pains generally. They begin their slow ascent in the afternoon, reach a zenith at night, then slowly descend till morning. The culminating point of these nightly headaches is variable.

Go on Forever, Unending Nightmare

- Very despondent, does not think he will ever get better.
- Dreams about his disease.
- Feeling as if going insane, or about to be paralyzed.
- Sensations: as if going insane; as if about to be paralyzed; of apathy and indifference.
- Terrible dread of night on account of mental and physical exhaustion when she awakes; it is intolerable, death is preferable; she fears to prepare for night and is positively in abject fear of suffering, in form of exhaustion on awaking.
- Always agg. as night approaches; leaves her about daylight, which she prays for.
- Attacks gradually get more severe and last longer.
- Crying infants, who begin crying immediately after birth.
- Syphilitic headache for many months, piercing, pressing excruciating over right eye.
- Deafness gradually increasing until she could scarcely hear at all.
- Complete deafness; nothing abnormal to be seen.
- Vomiting for weeks or months.
- Total loss of appetite for months, little or nothing satisfies him.
- Obstinate constipation for years.
- Yellow offensive leucorrhœa, watery or not, so profuse it daily soaks through napkins and runs to heels of stockings and on her feet.
- Aching of genitals, could not sit still for over a month.
- Pains in muscles of loins, terrible to bear, preventing sleep and forcing him to cry out.
- Constant pain across small of back.
- Hard cough, agg. at night, when it is continuous, preventing sleep.
- Chronic asthma... with great anguish and inability to retain a recumbent position.
- Attacks of spasmodic bronchial asthma for 25 years. The attack would come on only at night after lying down, or during a thunderstorm, and produces the most intense insomnia, entirely preventing sleep for days and nights together.
- Terrific pain by night; for five months, every night most intense neuralgic pains.
- Pain in lower extremities, excruciating, completely banish sleep.
- Great restlessness at night, impossible to keep long in one position.
- Absolute sleeplessness.
- Wakes soon after midnight and cannot sleep again till 6 AM.
- During the whole 24 hours can only rest from 8 to 10 AM.
- Absolute sleeplessness for 11 to 14 days and nights.
- Total loss of sleep for 22 successive days and night.
- Tendency to heavy drinking; alcoholism.
- Craving alcohol, in any form. Hereditary tendency to alcoholism.
- An old gentleman has had for some years cancer on right malar bone; no rest, his agony excruciating in extreme.

The head pains are maddening, and are accompanied by great restlessness, sleeplessness and nervous excitement. Headaches, like the hand-washing, may precede epileptic fits. These intense neuro-psychological concomitants suggest that unravelling the essential nature of the Syphilinum headaches may provide a key to perceiving the inner mental and emotional state.

Syphilinum is well known for its linear headaches. Lines of pain may extend from eyes to occiput. Pains run in a line from temple to temple or from brain centre to vertex, forming an inverted letter T. As there are no linear configurations in the brain, it is obvious that these pains are not following any anatomical structure. This suggests a neuro-illogical, strange, and highly characteristic phenomenon and implies that the line is an important component of Syphilinum's inner nature.

We should therefore consider the nature of lines. Straight lines are generated by pure light or are man made.

> Laser beams travel in direct lines. They are sterile, bearing no life.
>
> Artificial canals cut a straight line. They are clinical, dead.

Nature, like her mother,
earth,
twists,
circles
and spirals. Rivers wind and
curve
as swirling turbulence
coils DNA into new life.

A light beam holds its linear course forever bright with unmanifested potential. Then it encounters a gravitational force, planet, sphere, black hole. Turning head, it whistles softly, spirals round as life begins. Long straight nerves convolute into brainy bundles, blood vessels twist and turn. Like the number 10, male and female, we are completed by a spiral composed of linear and circular motions.

Cannot Converge

- Arithmetical calculations difficult.
- Great difficulty, and sometimes impossibility, of concentrating the thoughts on particular subjects.
- Tongue turns to one side when protruded; difficulty in mastication, cannot turn food with tongue so readily from right to left as in other direction.
- Strabismus paralyticus, the rectus internus being involved, and the eye turning outward.
- Hungry but could eat nothing but fluids, as mastication was impossible.
- Singular feeling as if teeth had all got out of place, and on closing jaws teeth do not come well together.
- Left ovary swollen, during coitus, at, moment of orgasm, a sharp, cutting pain like a knife.
- Head; open fontanels (C)
- Chest; xiphoid process absent (C)

Converging to a Point, Triangles

- Always washing the hands.
- Throbbing in temples and ears, boring in ears meeting in center of brain.
- Headache through temples, thence vertically like an inverted letter T.
- Syphilitic headache for many months, piercing, pressing, extending deep into brain.
- Lancinating pain in occiput.
- Large prominent spot on center of forehead.
- Red papulous eruption round left inner canthus.
- Itching of left inner canthus.
- Pain in right inner canthus as if blood went there and could go no further.
- Lids inflamed, esp. at outer canthus.
- On waking, gum in right canthus.
- Agglutination of lids. Both eyes glued in morning.
- During sleep lids adhere; in infantile syphilis.
- Strabismus paralytica, eye turning inward, and pupil can only be turned outward as far as median line.
- On turning eye to left feels momentary coldness in inner half of right eye.
- Pimples became confluent where they were most dense.
- Intense earache in right ear, incisive pains thrusting into ear.
- Tongue thickly coated, dirty, edges indented or serrated by teeth.
- Two large ulcers... (sensation) cut down as with a knife.
- Septum of nose threatened.
- Single small lunae cleft in upper incisors, permanent set, which incisors are dwarfed in their general dimensions, and converge at their tips.

But where are the circles in liney Syphi-linum? Long bones bow and curve, rounded spines bend, worm-like sensations wriggle, eruptions are circumscribed, mucus is ball shaped.

Syphi-linum has separated line from curve, male from female, 1 from 0. Like a laser beam traversing an endless universe, these lines yearn to coil.
Lonely linear,
loves travel,
desperately seeking gravid gravity,
birth and death, black hole or centre brain.

If the notion of an endless line seems like a nightmare, there is more to come in Syphilinum. The following symptom holds a key to this remedy as well as the syphilitic miasm.

Constant linear headache, commencing at both angles of forehead and extending in <u>parallel lines</u> backward - a precursor of epileptic attack.

What is the essence of parallel lines? The definition is this: These lines can never meet. Never. Ever. Ever… Ever. Not from here till everlasting eternity will they find each other. Doomed to travel an endless, lifeless path, without so much as a curve, a spiral, a bend, a kiss. Syphilitic nightmare, no conjunction, no termination, no stereophonic oneness. Perpetual parallel rays of cursing sun, no grace of night to end this day. Imagine 11 to 22 nights of incessant torturous insomnia. Imagine splitting headaches lasting for months, left right brain in parallel plight. Imagine maddening pains driving insane, slow to grow and slow to go. Imagine the anguished despair of an endless disease stretching far into an eternal future. A personal hell composed of a single thought - there is no end!

Every long day is blessed with a night, every long night is kissed by a dawn. Imagine the feeling of no gentle end, no sweet sleep, just prolonged forever. Then Syphilinum can have but one wish, one prayer - please dear God let it end. Please let me die of death or love or pain or birth. Let me meet someplace, somewhere, in the centre brain, in the here and now, let me sleep, let me unite, let me converge!

- Children's teeth are cupped.
- Teeth decaying at edge of gum and breaking off.
- First central upper incisors serrated, permanent teeth point towards each other, inner side concave; edges serrated.
- Teeth; stick together, as if glued (C)
- Teeth pain amel. pressing teeth together.
- Rectum seems tied up with strictures; when enemate were used the agony of passage was like labor.
- Pricking in chancre, as though punctured by pins.
- Sharp zigzag shooting pains in region of uterus.
- Left ovary swollen, during coitus, at moment of orgasm, a sharp cutting pain like a knife.
- Pain and oppression at bifurcation of bronchia.
- Choking sensation from fauces to bifurcation of bronchia, great mental distress.
- Oppression of chest to such an extent as to almost arrest breathing; asthma caused by sensation as if sternum were being gradually drawn towards dorsal vertebra.
- Pain in center of chest as if skin were drawn up, on drawing the head back.
- Lancinating pain in heart at night, from base to apex. (from apex to base, Med.)
- Pain in coccyx at its junction with sacrum.
- Caries of cervical spine with great curvature in same region, directly forward, occiput sinking down to a level with it and resting on protuberance of curvature.
- Pains in muscles of loins, generally in left, sharp, cutting spasms.
- Pedunculated pin-head warts on neck.
- Rheumatism at insertion of deltoid, agg. from raising arm laterally.
- Right second finger is swollen and stiffened.
- Osteosarcoma in center of right tibia.
- All the flexors seem to become contracted and shortened.
- Contracted, painful feeling in soles, as if tendons were too short.
- Sharp rheumatic pain, burning like fire, in left side of right instep and below inner malleolus, prevents her from moving foot agg. when toe is pointed inward.
- Extremities; tied, as if; lower limbs (C)
- Skin; eruptions; crusty; conical (C)
- Darting pains in irregular attacks.
- Prickly sensation as if the numb parts were punctured by a great number of needles.
- Pains like sawing off his bones with a dull saw.
- Though 17 looked 12, was so reduced and dwarfed.
- Dwarfed, shrivelled-up, old-looking babies and children.
- Amelioration in the mountains.

Parallel lines,
equal signs, cannot complete
mathematical sums. Parallel footprints,
space and time, man and woman can't be one.
Parallel cracks, both sides of tongue, present moment never comes. Cutting pains
prevent a climax; never experience sexual oneness. Symmetrical eruptions, jaws can't
meet, must wash hands, binding feet.

Infants born in dire despair, parallel posterity stretching ahead.
Lonesome agony, sterile existence, screaming, begging, let us meet.
On the peak of a mountain, let us meet. Crest of a tibia, let us meet.
Apex of deltoid, zenith of heart, septum of nose, let us meet.
Saw-like pains, lightning strikes,
jagged teeth, longest night,
inner canthus, self
destruct;
parallel
end.

- Aggravation electric storms.
- Irritable, excited, walking much of the time, does not want to be soothed, violent on being opposed, has tremors, seems on the verge of convulsions, dazed, absent-minded, **always washing her hands**.

Time Converging to a Point

- Pains commence at 2 PM, gradually increasing till they reach their **acme** at 9 PM, continuing exceedingly acute till 3 or 4 AM, subsiding with daybreak.
- The pains gradually increase and decrease; they get worse at 4 or 5 PM, **attain their height** at 2 or 3 AM, ceasing about 8 AM.
- Headache, neuralgic in character, causing sleeplessness and delirium at night; commencing at 4 PM; worse from 10 to 11 and ceasing at daylight.
- Neuralgic headache causing sleeplessness or delirium at night, always commencing about four PM; agg. from 10 to 11 PM, and ceasing at daylight.
- Pains commence about 4 PM, **culminate** about midnight in delirium, and cease entirely at daylight.
- Syphilitic iritis, intense pain steadily increasing night after night; agg. between 2 and 5 AM, **coming almost at the minute** and ceasing same way.
- Neuralgia every night, beginning about 8 or 9 PM, gradually increasing in severity until it **reached its height** about 3 or four AM, and after continuing thus for two or three hours, gradually decreased and finally ceased about 10 AM.

Loss Of Present

- Loss of memory.
- Loss of memory: cannot remember names of books, persons or places.
- Loses remembrance of passing occurrences, names, dates, etc. while all occurrences previous to inception of disease are remembered as distinctly as ever, almost without effort.
- Great difficulty, and sometimes impossibility, of concentrating the thoughts on particular subjects; yet at the same time can recollect consecutive events and details which occurred 25 or 30 years previously in the order of occurrence, almost without effort.
- Losing continuity of thought and memory; makes repeated mistakes in figures.

Dream

I took Syphilinum 1M. Within an hour I felt as if I was coming down with a whopper of a cold - sore throat, runny nose, grumpy mood. Got into a hot bath and then bed. Had a few weird dreams, one which came right on the heels of taking the remedy:

I was going to a concert in a place where I went to folk concerts in the mid-1950's. I had a time machine, and I was going back to re-experience it. I also was looking to see if I could spot myself, knowing that me at 15 wouldn't recognise me at 54. And there I was – I was wearing a serving tray on my head and it had two points – like horns – coming out of the top surface.

WW

Play

Mr. YY:	Hi honey, how was your day?
Mrs. XX:	Did you deliver the letters I asked you to?
Mr. YY:	It was really stressful at the office today.
Mrs. XX:	They were quite important. I hope they get there in time.
Mr. YY:	The boss was unhappy with the unification project.
Mrs. XX:	Hmmm… I should get some dinner.
Mr. YY:	He said I would have to re-do it with Miss XY.
Mrs. XX:	How about pizza?
Mr. YY:	I can't stand working with her. She just can't seem to follow the same line of thought as me.
Mrs. XX:	Pizza and burgers. Do you think that will work together?
Mr. YY:	Maybe. Are you day shift or night shift next week?
Mrs. XX:	If you have work to finish, I'll watch TV after dinner. ... Day shift.
Mr. YY:	Oh well, I'm night shift. Guess we won't be seeing each other much. It makes the week seem so long.
Mrs. XX:	I do hope those letters get there in time. The post takes forever these days.

Syphilinum Synthesis

Verb

Sensation:
Parallel lines that never meet, stretching on forever.

Function:
Must converge to a point.

Form:
Parallel lines. Triangle

Image

No present; parallel past and future do not converge in the now.
No union; parallel male and female separated by sexual disease.
Immediate pleasure resulting in endless despair.

Q.E.D

Thallium

Toxicological Information

Second to pure provings, toxicological data is the most rewarding source of symptoms in our remedies. It is interesting to note that much of the information in our materia medica comes directly from poisonings. Especially useful are reports of organic pathology that do not arise in provings. In the past this information was gathered diligently from medical journals, books, personal accounts and herbal medicine.

Now that we live in the "information super-highway" age of computers, a vast amount of toxicological data has become available. It is our duty to tap in to this unlimited source of symptoms so as to enrich our materia medica. This information can stand alone or be added to proving symptoms to form a complete picture. Once collected, the data should be arranged according to the homoeopathic schema and converted into repertory language.

Much of this toxicological information is a result of the extreme misery that humankind has inflicted on itself. Drugs, pesticides, radiation – all have caused disease, pain and suffering. All the more so when these poisonings have been used with malicious intent, as in the case of Thallium. As homœopaths we possess the power to convert poisonous lead into the golden knowledge needed to heal our planet.

JS

Thallium

Characteristics

Thallium is a bluish-white metal first discovered by William Crookes in 1861. It sits between mercury and plumbum in the 6th period of the Periodic Table. In nature thallium occurs in trace amounts in the form of salts and is found with many of the earth crust heavy metals, especially copper, gold, silver, antimony, bismuth, barium, zinc and cadmium. Commercially it is extracted from lead; however, the United States and many other countries no longer produce thallium.

Thallium takes its name from the Greek, *thallos* (green bud) because it produces a green line on spectral analysis. Chemically it resembles both lead and aluminium and often combines with bromine, chlorine, fluorine and iodine.[1]

Uses

The first application of thallium was as a medicine to treat night sweats in tuberculosis patients and as a topical salve for ringworm; later it was a therapy for syphilis, gonorrhoea, gout and dysentery.[2] When it became apparent that thallium was a potent toxin, it was used worldwide as rat, ant and cockroach poison. The United States banned thalllium as a pesticide in 1965.

Today thallium is primarily used in the semiconductor industry and in the manufacture of photocells, infrared detectors and fireworks. Because of its refractory ability, thallium is a component in the production of optical glass, coloured glass and imitation precious stones, which sparkle from the presence of thallium. In extremely cold climates it is used as an anti-freeze in mercury thermometers. Doctors employ thallium in cardiac scanning tests, injecting a small amount of a radioactive thallium isotope into the blood, where it replaces potassium and attaches itself to the heart muscle.

Environmental Presence

Most of the thallium in the environment enters as a byproduct of coalburning power plants, smelting operations and cement factories. Thallium may be inhaled, eaten or absorbed through the skin by those living near cement factories and other industrial operations or near hazardous waste sites containing thallium. It pollutes water by leaching from ore processing operations. From the water thallium is consumed by fish and shellfish and from the soil it is absorbed by plants, such as food crops and tobacco.[1]

Repertory of Toxicology Symptoms of Thallium Salts:

(NR) – New Rubric

Mind

Agitation
Anger, violent
Apathy
Aphasia
Concentration difficult
Confusion of mind
Confusion of mind when spoken to
Delirium
Delusions, voices, hears
Delusions, poisoned
Fight desires to
Irritability
Irritability from noise
Lies, makes up stories to fill memory gaps (NR)
Loquacity
Memory, weakness of
Memory, weakness of, remembers names
Mistakes, makes in calculating
Mood, changeable emotional lability
Rage
Rage, violent
Restlessness
Slowness
Speech, incoherent
Starting from noise, violently
Striking
Unconsciousness

Head

Hair falling
Hair gray, becomes
Inflammation of brain

Vertigo

Sitting,
Staggering with
Rising, on

Nose

Discoloration, redness, saddle

Face

Chewing motion of the jaw
Eruptions, herpes
Eruptions, pustules
Eruptions, cheeks
Eruptions, rash
Paralysis, facial nerves, peripheral nerves, 1st and 8th cranial nerves not affected (NR)

Eye

Atrophy of optic nerve
Cataract
Falling of lids
Hair falling from brows, except inner third portion (see Skin, hair falls out)
Hair falling from eyelashes (see Skin, hair falls out)
Inflammation, optic nerve
Inflammation, lids
Inflammation, conjunctiva

Occupational exposure is the most common route to thallium toxicity, followed by ingesting food or rat poison and smoking tobacco contaminated with thallium. Its reputation as a colourless, tasteless, toxic element is well known by criminals and many accounts of murder by thallium poisoning appear in literature. Agatha Christie uses thallium as the effective assassin in her novel, *The Pale Horse*. The film, "The Young Poisoner's Handbook," chronicles the true story of a young chemist who poisons his co-workers with the deadly metal.[3]

Political Use

Thallium has been a ruthless agent in biological civil warfare. The South African Truth and Reconciliation Commission, investigating atrocities during the apartheid era, discovered that the government had run a covert biological and chemical warfare program to assassinate black anti-apartheid activists.[4] Army scientists testified to the Commission about their plans to render Nelson Mandela unable to lead the ANC by poisoning him with thallium shortly before his release from prison.[5]

The government of Iraq has been criticised by world human rights organisations for its flagrant use of thallium to annihilate political adversaries. Since 1980 Amnesty International, the United Nations Commission on Human Rights and other human rights groups have issued numerous reports of thallium poisoning of thousands of Shiite Kurds and hundreds of dissident Iraqi soldiers and opposition party members. [6, 7, 8]

In 1980 three political suspects were poisoned while being held in Iraqi prison; two were released and evacuated to the UK, where one died and the other recovered. A third prisoner was fed thallium tainted food the day before her release from prison. That day she developed nausea, and before she died, paralysis of limbs, inability to swallow, respiratory insufficiency and alopecia.[9] Iraq's chief architect, who "had extensive knowledge about the construction of Saddam's palaces, tunnels, and bunkers," was killed with thallium. The head of Iraq's leading university, long a political activist, was poisoned by thallium, but because he was outside of a government controlled area, was treated medically and survived. Two former Iraqi security directors are suspected to have died from thallium toxicity.[10]

In 1993 a member of the British House of Commons reported, "As we spoke, 300 people were entering Tehran from Iraq. They had been released from prison, which was astonishing. They had served 10, 11 or 12 years – we must remember that Saddam Hussein took control in 1979. Later in the week, they began to die because, as they left prison, they had been given thallium injections. To have hope dashed so cruelly is unbelievable."[11] Iraqi exiles living in London have recounted a number of poisonings and deaths from thallium-laced food and beverages surreptitiously administered by undercover Iraqi agents based in the U.K. [12]

Eyes; inflammation; pigmentary, retinitis pigmentosa
Eyes; inflammation; pigmentary, resembles beaten metal (NR)
Movement, eyeballs, constant, involuntary
Movement, eyeballs, constant, rolling movement, up and down
Paralysis of muscles of eyeball
Paralysis of optic nerve, amaurosis
Photophobia
Pupils, dilated
Redness
Strabismus
Turned, upward

Vision
Vision, blurred
Vision, dim
Vision, dim, right eye
Vision loss of, blindness
Vision loss of, blindness, colors for

Mouth
Cracked
Discoloration, gums, blue line on margin
Discoloration, gums, purple (NR)
Dryness
Motion, tongue, difficult
Odor, offensive
Salivation
Speech, difficult
Inflammation
Taste, disturbance of (NR)

Throat
Swallowing, difficult

Stomach
Appetite wanting
Inflammation
Nausea
Pain, cramping
Pain, cutting
Vomiting
Vomiting, blood

Abdomen
Pain, cramping

Rectum
Diarrhea
Constipation
Involuntary stool

Stool
Bloody

Bladder
Retention of urine

Urine
Albuminous
Bloody

Genitalia – Female
Menses, absent, amenorrhea

Larynx
Voice, weak

Respiration
Respiration, difficult

Chest
Inflammation, bronchial tubes
Pain, heart
Oedema, pulmonary
Inflammation, lungs

Toxicology

Biological effects

In the human body thallium mimics potassium and localises especially in the heart and the pigmented tissues of the eye.[13] Muscular and cardiac symptoms are created as thallium replaces potassium, depolarises membranes in the nerves and heart and antagonises the effect of calcium on the heart.[14] When a potassium source, such as orange juice, is ingested, the symptoms are aggravated.[15]

A study of children born to parents who ate thallium contaminated food indicates an increase in congenital malformations.[16] It is known that thallium can cross blood-brain and placental barriers and has a half life of one month in the human body.[1]

Animal studies report testicular absorption in male rats and congenital malformations, especially of the bones. One rat study showed demylelination of the dorsal root ganglia.[14]

Initial toxic effects

The initial effects of thallium poisoning appear in 4 to 48 hours and are felt in the digestive organs with excessive salivation, violent abdominal pain, nausea and haemorrhage with bloody vomiting and bloody diarrhoea.[17] Within 5 to 10 days alopecia occurs leading to complete loss of body hair in one month. Alopecia is unique to thallium poisoning and is characterised first by hair being plucked easily from the head. Later, it comes out by handfuls, beginning with the scalp and pubis, then axillae and face. An odd symptom is retention of the medial third part of the eyebrows or 'signe de sourcil.'[3] Dark pigmentation develops under the scalp in the roots of the hair, and also is apparent in the hair shaft prior to the onset of alopecia.[14]

Neurological Symptoms

Thallium causes severe affliction of the central, peripheral and autonomic nervous systems, including optic neuritis, ataxia, tremors, paresthesia and paralysis of lower extremities. Sensory nerves are more strongly affected than motor neurons and lower limbs are more seriously involved than upper. Within one week, pain and tenderness develop in the legs, worsening until even the slightest movement becomes almost unbearable. There is burning pain in the soles of the feet.[14] The lower limbs suffer extreme sensitivity and severe burning pain from the lightest touch, and this sensitivity and pain ascend to the abdomen and chest. Stabbing pain in the lower limbs and abdomen is likened to the severe pain of tabes dorsalis, which, Clarke reports, has been relieved by potentised thallium. Neuralgic pain in the toes, feet and legs is described as "lightening like."[18] A general hyperirritability, especially to sound, can cause the thallium poisoned patient to jump violently.[15]

Extremities

Contraction of muscles and tendons
Convulsion, upper limbs
Discoloration, fingers, nails, white striae, broad band shaped stripes (Mee's lines) (NR)
Eruptions, pustules
Eruptions, rash
Eruptions, upper limbs, pustules
Eruptions, upper limbs, rash
Eruptions, hand, purple
Eruptions, hand, pustules
Eruptions, hand, rash
Eruptions, fingers, rash
Eruptions, lower limbs,
Eruptions, lower limbs, pustules,
Motion, involuntary
Motion, loss of power of
Numbness, hand
Numbness, foot
Pain, burning, hand
Pain, burning, foot
Pain, burning, foot, sole
Pain, burning, foot, toes, first
Pain, general, lower limbs, muscles
Pain, joints, wandering
Pain, lower limbs, extending upwards
Pain, lower limbs, legs and feet, extending to thighs, abdomen and anterior chest (NR)
Pain; foot, soles, lighting, like
Pain; toes, first, lighting, like
Pain, toes first, neuralgic
Pain, knee neuralgic
Pain thigh, neuralgic
Pain, leg neuralgic
Pain, foot
Pain, neuralgic
Paralysis
Paralysis, ascending
Perspiration, hand
Perspiration, foot
Position, sense of, decreased (NR)
Prickling
Reflexes increased
Sensitive
Sensitive, palm
Sensitive, fingers
Sensitive, finger, tips
Sensitive, leg, tibia
Sensitive, foot
Sensitive, foot, sole
Sensitive, toes
Stiffness
Stiffness, joints,
Stiffness, lower limbs, knee
Stiffness, lower limbs, ankle
Tingling, hand, painful
Tingling, thigh, painful
Tingling, foot, painful extremities
Tottering
Twitching (see Generalities)
Weakness
Weakness, lower limbs
Weakness, foot, paralytic
Weakness, paralytic

Sleep

Comatose
Sleeplessness
Sleepiness, overpowering

Perspiration

Perspiration
Profuse
Scanty
Single parts

Thallium toxicity affects the eyes, producing optic nerve inflammation and pseudo retinitis pigmentosa. On examination, the optic disc is swollen and its pigmentation resembles beaten metal.[19] Lids and conjunctiva may be inflamed. Vision may be fuzzy and dim, with misjudgement of distance and loss of colour vision. The muscles of the eyeball are affected resulting in strabismus, involuntary up and down movements or paralysis due to the destruction of the oculomotor nerve.[14]

The facial nerve is inflamed and paralysed, with falling of the eyelids.[17] Numbness and tingling of the hands and feet are experienced. Exaggerated reflexes of the legs and arms are followed by decreased nerve conduction and paresis in the extremities.[14] Ataxia and vertigo interfere with walking. Some victims have reported less ability to sense the position of their limbs.[3] Paralysis begins in the lower limbs ascending to upper extremities and to the respiratory and deglutition muscles, a progression similar to Guillain-Barre syndrome. All sorts of tremblings, twitchings, chorea and convulsions distress the person with thallium toxicity.

Thallium's disturbance in the autonomic nervous system is evident by episodes of orthostatic hypotension, labile blood pressure, urinary retention, persistant constipation, salivary gland dysfunction causing salivation and then dryness of the mouth and cardiac arrhythmias. Cardiac arrhythmias often lead to death.[14]

Other Symptoms

Herpes or pustules erupt on the face and fissures open at the corners of the mouth. Gums have a bluish or purplish line as in lead poisoning. Profuse sweating followed by destruction of the sweat glands results in dry, scaly skin.[14] White spots in the shape of half-moons or streaks (Mee's lines), mark the nails of the fingers and toes.[3]

If a large quantity or continuous repetition of thallium is administered, alopecia persists and perilous systemic symptoms appear; hypertension, changes in heart electrocardiography, sinus tachycardia, hypokalemia, leukocytosis and thrombocytopenia. Many patients develop aphasia, progressive paresis and paralysis, total or one-sided.[3] Convulsions and coma often precede death. Postmortem examinations reveal damage to eye, liver, kidney, intestinal and testicular tissues.[1]

Mental Symptoms

The mental and emotional symptoms of thallium poisoning progress rapidly to serious levels. Patients are talkative, often irrationally, and may have difficulty with calculations. Many experience narcolepsy or sleeplessness. Restlessness and hysteria appear along with delirium and hallucinations, psychosis and severe dementia. Often patients have memory lapses, both

Skin

Burning, touch, on
Dry
Ecchymoses
Electric sparks as of, from, sensation
Eruptions, acne
Eruptions, herpetic
Eruptions, pustular
Eruptions, rash, purple (NR)
Eruptions; urticaria, hives; clothing, from pressure of
Eruptions; urticaria, hives; any pressure (dermatographia) (NR)
Hair falls out shedding of hair in tufts, handfuls, pubic, axillary, eyebrows and lashes, except medial 3rd part of eyebrows (NR) (see Generalaties)
Numbness
Prickling, tingling
Rough
Sensitiveness

Generalities

Chorea
Convulsions
Convulsions, clonic (see Extremities)
Convulsions, epileptic
Digitalis poisoning, antidotes
Emaciation
Food, orange juice agg (NR)
Hair falling, (see Skin)
Inflammation, general, nerves
Lassitude
Night
Pain, as from burning
Pain; general; appearing suddenly
Sudden manifestations
Paralysis
Paralysis, one sided, left
Potassium agg (NR)
Pressure agg
Pulse, frequent
Pulse, slow
Relaxation of muscles
Sensitiveness, externally
Shocks, sensations; electric, like
Sluggishness of the body
Touch agg
Touch slight, agg
Trembling, externally
Twitching
Weakness

long and short term. One patient with memory loss convincingly lied about events to fill in the missing gaps.[14]

ANTIDOTE

Medical treatment for thallium poisoning is Prussian blue, potassium ferric ferrocyanide. Thallium binds with this chelating agent in the intestines, probably by replacing potassium, and is excreted in the stool.[20] In some cases potassium chloride is given intravenously, although it seems to worsen the brain symptoms during treatment.[21] Also useful is milk thistle (Silybum marianum), which is recognized as having protective properties for the liver.[22]

Cases

CASE 1

A *Lancet* article describes the onset of thallium toxicity in a 19-month-old girl. Her illness began with a high fever and a major convulsion. Over the next 3 days she became increasingly clumsy and lethargic and developed slurring of her speech. By the seventh day she was unable to sit, stand or walk, and had difficulty with swallowing. The following day she had another generalised convulsion lasting about 5 minutes. The child also started losing hair, which typically occurs 10-15 days after thallium ingestion.[23]

CASE 2

In December, 1994, a female Chinese university student complained of persistent abdominal pain with episodes of colic. A few days later her hair began to fall out and she had constipation and delayed menses. Within 5 days the young woman was bald and after a month she had total alopecia, except for the inner third of her eyebrows. During this time the patient was hospitalised and treated with traditional Chinese medicine. The alopecia reversed and she returned to university.

Within a few weeks, unknowingly exposed to thallium again, the student felt pain in her hands and feet, joints and muscles; and had dysphonia, vertigo, blurred vision and intermittent upward staring of her eyes. Colour vision disappeared and all colours appeared white. Her condition worsened rapidly with intensified vertigo and tremors and oculogyric crisis – her eyeballs rolled and became fixed in an extreme position. She developed facial nerve palsy, poor muscle coordination and hypersensitivity in a "glove and sock-like distribution." Deep tendon reflexes in the lower extremities were reduced, while upper extremities remained normal. The slightest pressure on her skin caused raised red lines to appear (dermatographia).

De Maupassant: "I've got the pox!. . . .the great pox, the one which Francis I died of. The majestic pox, pure and simple; the elegant syphilis. . . I've got the pox. . .and I am proud of it, by thunder, and to hell with the bourgeoisie. Allelujah, I've got the pox, so I don't have to worry about catching it any more, and I screw the street whores and trollops, and afterwards I say to them 'I've got the pox.' They are afraid and I just laugh."

History of Syphilis

The patient developed bulbar palsy, respiratory distress due to central nervous system disturbance and involuntary chewing movements of her mouth. Spasms of both upper limbs stiffened her arms and raised them involuntarily above her body. She became blind. Consciousness ranged from restlessness to drowsiness and then into coma with convulsive movements of the arms and fixed staring of the eyes. Coma and weakened respiration set in two weeks after her second contact with thallium.

Similar to many survivors of thallium poisoning, this patient had a slow recovery with persisting symptoms. Five years later, numerous neurological abnormalities remain. Her vision is greatly diminished, but she can perceive colours and recognise people from one metre away. Short term memory and memory of events is impaired, although basic math and verbal skills have returned. Unable to speak clearly, she understands most of what is said to her. Respiratory support is required. She is generally bedridden, although able to lift her hands, move her legs, sit without assistance and stand for a few minutes.[24, 25]

Case 3

A male victim of thallium poisoning was admitted to hospital with undiagnosed heart pain, followed three weeks later by general malaise, unsteady walking and a pustular rash on his legs and hands. By that time he had become confused and disoriented and had developed vomiting, pronounced alopecia and a purplish rash on his hands and fingers. Nystagmus, facial muscle weakness, and weakness of his limbs were present. The man's movement was coordinated but slow, and his sense of joint position was reduced. Due to ataxia, he walked with a wide gait.

After treatment the patient was followed by the neuropsychology department. Four years later chronic peripheral neuropathy continued. Although muscle power had increased and his gait was less wide, generally his motion was slow. His memory remained impaired. Notably, the man's normal psychological state had changed. "He was irritable and had aggressive outbursts. He impulsively and remorselessly assaulted members of his family and menaced people in the street. He lost his temper with a neighbour, whom he alleged had poisoned him." None of these behaviours was present before the thallium intoxication.[26]

See Appendix B for references.

Consumptions sow
In hollow bones of man! strike their sharp shins,
And mar men's spurring. Crack the lawyer's voice
That he may never more false title plead,
Nor sound his quillets shrilly; hoar the flamen,
That scolds against the quality of flesh
And not believes himself; down with the nose,
Down with it flat; take the bridge quite away
Of him that, his particular to forsee,
Smells from the general weal; make curled-pate ruffians bald;
And let the unscarred braggarts of the war
Derive some pain from you; Plague all,
That your activity may defeat and quell
The source of all erection. There's more gold;
Do you damn others, and let this damn you,
And ditches grave you all!

Shakespear, *"Timon of Athens"*

Thallium Synthesis

Verb

Sensation:
Electric shock.

Function:
Atrophy.

Sensation and function:
Exaggerated reflexes followed by decreased nerve conduction and paresis. Violent over-stimulation leading to decay.

Strange symptom:
Complete loss of all body hair with retention of the medial third part of the eyebrows.

Totally exposed except for innermost self.

Image

Attacked, hunted and poisoned by strict regime; dictator, defiance, dissident, fugitive.

From its history we find the abuse of thallium by totalitarian regimes wishing to get rid of political adversaries (Iraqi dissidents, Mandela). As a slow but powerful poison, thallium mimics natural pathology and is difficult to detect. In this way Thallium is extremely similar to Plumbum, which has delusions that he is persecuted and about to be poisoned or assassinated.

Jan Scholten has confirmed the opposite side of this picture by indicating that this remedy is suitable to ailing dictators and rulers who are losing control over their country, organisation or family. They try to prevent further erosion of their power by strictly enforcing of the old rules and by killing off the opposition.

A case from Vithoulkas is of a man suffering paralysis and atrophy. As a young boy he was frequently beaten by his father with a belt, yet he hid under the table and remained defiant.

Iridium to Plumbum

The Syphilitic Zone

The Periodic Shuffle

Delivering the promise
Iridium child of heaven,
radiates angelic light
which prisms into seven

She leaves half-sister Platina
confined by her division,
to step into stepmother's house
with laughter and derision

While old King Aurum, sadly
grasps his golden crown,
and yearns for unattainables
on the long climb down,

commanding General Mercury,
messenger on wings:
repulse the enemy without,
cause tyranny within,

force poor Thallium's dissident
to gross emaciation,
with torture and electric shocks
deep degeneration,

While Plumbum the dull fugitive
evades assassination,
by fleeing from lead bullets and
avoiding toxication,

And in the shelter Bismuth
devoid of all protection,
clings tightly to his mother
feeling very threatened

by the shadow of his
nuclear neighbour,
deep underground,
stalking shades of dead at night
hunting with his hound

So take me back Iridium
seven times eleven,
colour Plumbum's heavy grey
with rainbows from the heaven,
kiss poor Thallium's balding head,
turn Mercury to mild,
heal Platina's division
cuddle Bismuth's child

Raise King Aurum's
self esteem,
turn him upside down,
to realise that
in his heart
lies the real crown

For every kingdom's
bound to fall
through Life's degeneration,
the only peace
lies in the noble
moment of mutation

From sunny Helium's
Neon sky,
To Argon's Peter Pan,
From Krypton stars
and Xenon beasts
to Radon's upright man,
and all the way
to Luciferium
deep below the ground,
between the breath
of night and day
a shaft of truth is found

Never changing ever still
pivot of true life,
until the moment comes to start
the periodic slide,
a sharp electric current
turns on the noble light,
illuminating dark desires
stillness into strife

Carbon mother
in her taxi
riding up the mound,
four arms clutching
her organics
one for every child;
Hydrogen, Nitrogen
Oxygen, big C,
it's relatives like Adamas
who make it clear to see;
the motto for us carbons is
it's all to do with me,
no matter your significance
but how you are perceived

Then all the way
up to Iridium
starts the weary climb,
if only we could realise
we're climbing upside down,
and driving grimly forward
via mirror in reverse,
with each electron we acquire
comes a blessed curse.
Like a moth
into a flame
proton takes a dive
the mirror that we're living through
reflects our own desire

To live life in the here and now
noble and upright,
let go that extra atom
see the other side,
expensive metals end in rust
elements decline,
it's not the outer
but our soul
that will forever shine.
It's not what we can gain in life
but what we leave behind,
while winding back to Hydrogen
the universal mind.

From Fracastoro's 'Syphilis'

FROM IRIDIUM TO PLUMBUM

"I myself remember having seen one of the Cenomani for where the river Oglio with waters from the Sebinus flows with its abundance past rich meadow-lands, a conspicuous youth, more gifted and more brilliant then any in Italy. Scarce adolescent he was in the flowering springtime of his youth, a man of parts through his wealth and ancestry, with a handsome frame as well. He loved taming a swift, galloping horse, or putting on a helmet and shining in embossed arms, or hardening his youthful body in strenuous wrestling, and harrying wild animals in the hunt, or outstripping deer. All the goddesses of the Oglio desired him, all the maidens of the Po, the Goddesses of the woods, and the maidens of the countryside, all sighed over the marriage they desired. Perhaps one who had been spurned called on the avenging powers above, not in vain, and moved by her prayers the divine will to pity. For the poor youth, too self-assured, unaware of these great dangers, was seized by this plague, more savage than there has been anywhere or than will ever be seen at any future time. Gradually that glistening springtime, that flower of this youth perished utterly, that vigour of mind: then the wasting sickness with its filthy scabs (sheer horror) covered his sorry limbs, and, deep within, his bones began to swell large with hideous abscesses. Ugly sores (ye gods have pity) began to devour his lovely eyes and his love of the holy light and to devour his nose, which was gnawed away, leaving a piercing wound. A brief interval, then finally the unlucky youth departed heaven's hateful breath and the light. For him the neighbouring Alps, for him the wandering rivers wept. For him all the Goddesses of the Oglio and the maidens of the Po wept, and the Goddesses of the woods and the maidens of the countryside. Lake Sebinus poured out laments from its deep flowing river.

Morose Saturn drove this plague over the wretched earth: Mars too no less cruel contributed his savagery, and set in motion the effects of their fatal conjunction."

Pangloss made answer in these terms:
"O my dear Candide, you must remember Pacquette, that pretty wench, who waited on our noble Baroness; in her arms I tasted the pleasures of Paradise, which produced these Hell torments with which you see me devoured. She was infected with an ailment, and perhaps has since died of it; she received this present of a learned Franciscan, who derived it from the fountainhead; he was indebted for it to an old countess, who had it of a captain of horse, who had it of a marchioness, who had it of a page, the page had it of a Jesuit, who, during his novitiate, had it in a direct line from one of the fellow adventurers of Christopher Columbus; for my part I shall give it to nobody, I am a dying man."
"O sage Pangloss," cried Candide, "what a strange genealogy is this! Is not the devil the root of it?"

Voltaire, *Candide*

Conclusion

Syphilis As If

Syphilis
as if,

Life went on forever,
in parallel persistence,
perpetual nights
watch pointless days
of tedious existence.

And endless minutes stretching on,
paralysing bore,
till death becomes
the only purpose
worthwhile living for.

Life contracting to a dot,
blood softening a brain,
madness circulating tabloids
driving us insane.

Buboes eating into flesh
daggers grinding bone,
sex makes love to violence
love lurks red light zones.

Reaper smiles his deadly grin
winks to horseman four,
let's hit the road with a spirochete
call for brother war.

Wield a sword of platinum
show the world who's best,
paint a scorpion on the flag
raise the eagle crest.

I'll touch your gums, burst your hearts
ulcerate your soul,
chancre for your small-pox,
sanity for gold.

Sail me back to Europe,
London, Paris, Rome,
I'll concentrate you into camps
melt your flesh to bone.

And in the dark of a crystal night
remember my true goal,
I'm just a valve for Psora, dear,
an AID to bring you home.

Let sunlight fertilise you
let your population grow,
I'll rot your roots in the dead of night
preventing overflow.

And when my period is full
transforming six to seven,
gold to lead,
lead to pluto
blow us all to heaven.

Syphilis
as if.

Syphilis Synthesis

Verb

Sensation:
Suppressed Psora = Unsuccessful union = Parallel lines which can never meet = Tedium.

Function:
Must converge to a point. Impure coition.

Form

Parallel lines. Triangle.

Noun

Nose. Tibia. Bone. Root. Knife. Heavy metal under the ground. Mountain. Night. Covert sexuality. Death. Devil.

Name

Syn – with. Phil – Love. Philus or Phila – lover.
Syphilis – With love or with lover.
Hog lover (Fracastoro)

Disease origins:

• Every acute disease is an attempt to resolve the chronic disease from which it originates. (*'Homœopathic Laws'*).
• Syphilis is an acute expression of chronic psora.
∴ And as such it is an attempt to resolve psora.
• The exciting cause of an acute disease is a natural similar of its chronic and a key to its understanding. (*'Homœopathic Laws'*)
∴ Therefore, the exciting cause of syphilis is a natural similar to psora.
∴ Therefore, the exciting cause of syphilis is a key to understanding psora, indicating its main susceptibility.
• The exciting cause of syphilis is impure coition.
∴ Therefore, the main susceptibility and essence of psora is the non-union or unholy (un-whole) union (internal and external) of male and female.

Image :

The knife. Metal converging to a point.

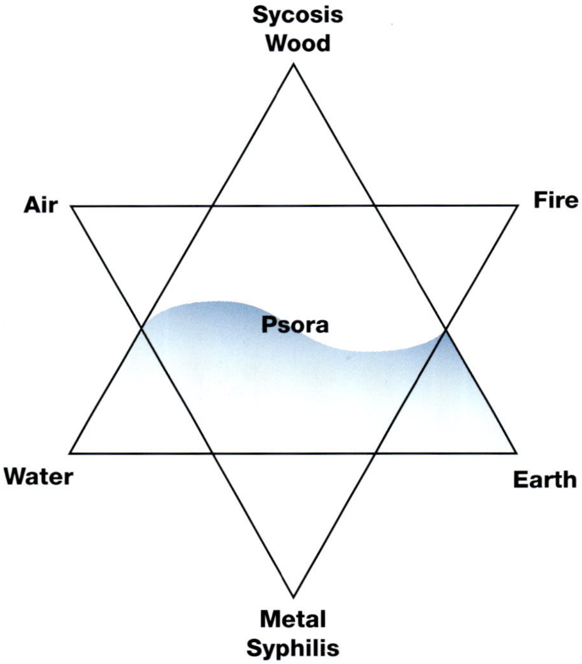
Sycosis
Wood
Air
Fire
Psora
Water
Earth
Metal
Syphilis

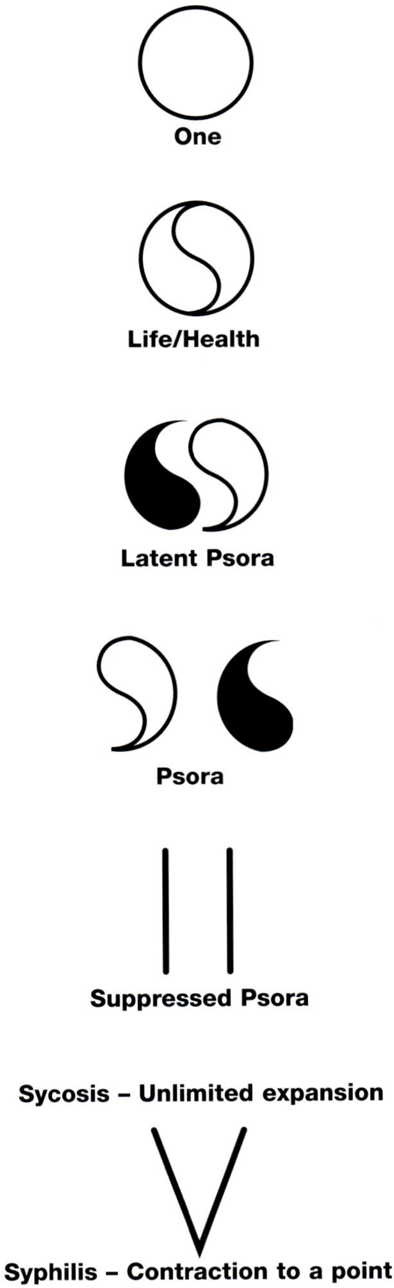
One
Life/Health
Latent Psora
Psora
Suppressed Psora
Sycosis – Unlimited expansion
Syphilis – Contraction to a point

Appendix A

Syphilis The Disease

From Fracastoro's 'Syphilis'

"...Olympus shook and trembled, the aether was contaminated by a discharge from the new disease. Gradually the tracts of the air and wide space received the plague, and an unusual putrefaction came into the empty air and carried contagion over all the sky, either because, so many stars being in conjunction with the burning Sun, the fiery power attracted many vapours from the earth and sea, which, mingled with the thin air and gripped by this new corruption, then brought a contagion very rarely seen; or something else, sent down from the aether above, tainted the realms of the air far and wide.

...It did not infect the silent creatures of the deep, the swarms of those that swim, nor birds, nor dumb animals wandering in high forests, nor herds of oxen or sheep or herds of horses, but out of all the species the one that is great through its mind, the human race, and it feeds, pasturing deep within our limbs. Moreover, from the whole of man this filthy disease seizes on that in the blood which is thick and dirty through its sluggishness, feeding on the rich slime. The disease and blood correspond in this particular way.

...What especially caused wonder was that even after the infection was caught the moon often completed its circle four times before sufficiently clear symptoms were shown. For it does not openly betray itself as soon as it has been received within a body, but it lies hid for a fixed period and gradually gains strength by feeding. Meanwhile, however, those afflicted were burdened by an unusual lethargy and, feeling a languor with no apparent cause, performed their tasks with increasing weariness and tried to keep themselves going although their whole body felt sluggish. Their natural liveliness fell downcast from their eyes, their colour from their unhappy brow. Slowly caries, born amid squalor in the body's shameful parts, became uncontrollable and began to eat the areas on either side and even the sexual organ. Then the symptoms of this defilement betrayed themselves more clearly. For as soon as the clean, kindly light of day had retreated and brought on the melancholy shades of night, and the innate heat, which at night usually makes for the deep internal parts, had abandoned the surface of the body, and no longer nursed the limbs now covered in a thick mass of humours, then the joints, arms, shoulder-blades and calves were tormented by intolerable pains. For when the contagion had passed through all the veins and had polluted even the humours and what was meant to feed the body, Nature whose wont is to reject what is harmful, attempted to expel the infected part from the whole

Modern Symptoms of Syphilis

INCUBATION	(3 wks to 3 months)
Diffusion through lymphatic system	
PRIMARY	(3 - 8 wks) (4 - 5 days later)
Chancre at point of inoculation; Usually round or oval, ulcerated, indurated, red, smooth, varnished surface. Secretes clear, serous fluid; painless; disappears in few weeks Local adenopathy Numerous hard, painless ganglions; persists for several months	
SECONDARY	(2 months to 3 yrs)
Cutaneous lesions: Roseola on thorax Diverse forms of papulous syphilides on palms and soles Painless, mucous lesions of mouth, genitals, anus Condylomata lata-papules at muco-cutaneous junctions Patches of alopecia Uveitis Papilledema Periostitis (bones and joints); aching pains in bones Visceral sx: hepatitis, kidney, spleen Malaise, headache, anorexia, nausea Meningitis, stiff neck Deafness	
LATENT	(Indefinite)
Fewer or more deceptive sx	

body towards the surface. But because this matter with its dense substance was slow and by reason of its sluggishness tenacious, much of it clung, during its passage to the nerves and muscles. Then as it spread it caused intolerable pains in the joints. This matter had a lighter element, more naturally inclined to erupt, which, as it was expelled, made for the surface of the skin and the limbs' extremities. Immediately unsightly sores broke out over all the body and made the face horrifyingly ugly, and disfigured the breast by their foul presence: the disease took on a new aspect: pustules with the shape of an acorn-cup and rotten with thick slime, which soon afterwards gaped wide open and flowed with a discharge like mucous and putrid blood. Moreover the disease gnawed deep and burrowed into the inmost parts, feeding on its victims' bodies with pitiable results: for on quite frequent occasions we ourselves have seen limbs stripped of their flesh and the bones rough with scales, and mouths eaten away yawn open in a hideous gape while the throat produced feeble sounds. As often either on the cherry or on Phyllis' mournful tree you have seen a thick fluid seep from the moist bark, then harden into a sticky gum, in just the same way, where this disease holds sway a mucus usually flows all over the body: then at last it solidifies into an ugly scab. So someone sighing over the springtime of his life and his beautiful youth, and gazing with wild eyes down at his disfigured members, his hideous limbs and swollen face, often in his misery railed against the Gods' cruelty, often against the stars. Meanwhile all the creatures on earth enjoyed the sweet slumbers of the weary and night's deep sleep; for the sufferers no rest was on hand, sleep had totally fled to the winds: for them Dawn as she blushed in her rising brought no pleasure: for them day was hostile, the night's apparition too was hostile. Ceres in none of her forms pleased them, none of Bacchus' gifts either, neither tasty banquets, nor abundance of good things, not the wealth of cities or of countryside, not any delight, however often they had sought out glittering streams, delightful valleys and gentle breezes on mountain tops. Prayers were showered upon the Gods, incense burned in their temples and their altars were decorated with rich gifts.

The Gods heard no prayers nor were moved by gifts."

TERTIARY
(5 to 10, 20, 30 yrs later)

Destructive cutaneous or sub-cutaneous gummas, of palate, nasal septum, pharynx, larynx, leg below knee, upper torso, face, scalp, tongue
Bone and joint lesions; deep boring pains
Gastric and hepatic lesions
Cardiovascular lesions; aortitis and aortic aneurysm or valve insufficiency
Meningovascular neurosyphilis:
- Dizziness
- Poor concentration
- Lassitude
- Insomnia
- Stiff neck
- Blurred vision
- Mental confusion
- Epileptiform seizures
- Papilledema
- Aphasia
- Hemiplegia
- Weakness and wasting of shoulder and arm muscles
- Spastic paraplegia
- Sudden transverse myelitis

Parenchymatous neurosyphilis:
- Insidious onset
- Tremors, convulsions
- Aphasia
- Hemiparesis
- Concentration difficult
- Memory weakness
- Hygiene deterioration
- Frequent weeping
- Temper tantrums
- Depression
- Delusions of grandeur
- Lack of insight
- Mutism
- Delusions: claim they are dead, blood has ceased to circulate, have no blood, body is utterly destroyed

Tabes dorsalis (locomotor ataxia)
- Lightning pain in legs
- Unsteadiness of gait, < dark
- Walks with feet wide apart
- Feeling of walking on foam rubber
- Hyperesthesia, paresthesia
- Loss of bladder sensation, urine retention, incontinence, infections
- Impotence
- Hallucinatory paranoia, confusion, dementia, agitation
- Delusions of persecution, of having committed crimes

(Merck Manual)

Syphilis: The Disease and its Influence

"... a disease which is so cruel, so distressing, so appalling that until now nothing so horrifying, nothing more terrible or disgusting, has ever been known on this earth".[1]

Appearance and Spread

Syphilis was a raging disease in the late 15th and early 16th centuries. In 1493 a significant outbreak occurred in Barcelona, which was recorded by a Spanish doctor who treated 20,000 victims. Some were members of Christopher Columbus's crew, who had just returned from their discovery voyage to Hispaniola. Throughout Spain, Columbus, his sailors and six visiting Arawaks were celebrating their triumphant voyage. "Sleeping with one of Columbus' sailors or one of the friendly Arawaks was like sleeping with the New World itself."[2] Disseminating rapidly from its initial appearance in Spain, the epidemic spread to Rome, France and beyond to Europe, Asia and Africa.

The rampage of syphilis can be traced on the map of military campaigns. In 1494 a Spanish military contingent entered Italy to assist in the defense of Naples, which was under attack by France. The invading French army of Charles VIII easily overcame the locals and their defenders and began months of debauched living among their captives. After withdrawing from Italy, the French mercenaries scattered to their homelands and to their unsuspecting loved ones, infecting all they met along the way in France, Switzerland and the Roman Empire. Within 10 years syphilis had worked its way across Europe.[1]

Attending the soldiers were prostitutes, who became both victims and reservoirs of the disease. Brothels, condoned by church and state, were popular local entertainment during the Renaissance. Their patrons suffered no shame.

> ... in every town there were fine public establishments... set up by royal order to preserve the honour of ladies... whence princes and bishops withdrew the girls they required ... seven hundred and eighteen girls [were] available to serve the council.... This single detail gives an idea of the rapidity with which the disease spread through each country.[1]

Ignorance by the public health officials and strong pecuniary interests of the brothel owners interfered with careful monitoring of the health of prostitutes. Whores and a liberal ethos hastened the distribution of syphilis. In the mid 1500s a Spanish physician treating syphilis in Lisbon, wrote, "It has caused so much damage that there is not a village in Europe with one hundred neighbours without ten of them dead of that ailment."[3]

Origins

Controversy and a variety of theories accompanied the European eruption of syphilis, known also as "the pox" or "bubas." From its beginning the disease was interpreted as God's wrath descended upon a morally impure people.[1] Astrologers, who understood epidemics based upon the placement of stars, claimed the cause was "the conjunction of Saturn (an unlucky planet) and Jupiter in the sign of the Scorpion and the house of Mars (also unlucky) on 25 November 1484.[1] Syphilis was first labeled the "French Disease" or "Morbus Gallus" by the Italians, although the French called it "the Neapolitan Disease."[1]

There are about three hundred examples of syphilitic neighbour-bashing: "the Spanish Disease," "the Castilian Disease," "the German Disease," "the Polish Disease," "the Arab Disease," "the Jewish Disease," "the Turkish Disease," "the Christian Disease," "the Ethiopian Disease," "the Ulcer of Canton," "the Chinese Disease" and "the Portuguese Disease."[2]

This "Great Imitator" of illnesses was the ambassador of blame as each country made its neighbour and enemy culpable for the destructive and loathsome affliction. A Spanish historian wrote, "... in truth [they] would have had the name better, if they called it the disease of the Indies."[2]

American Origin

Medical historians believe that syphilis was contracted first from the Arawak Indians in the West Indies, where a similar, but benign, form of the treponema had long been endemic.[1] When the crew members of Columbus came in contact, casually or intimately, with the mild skin symptoms of the Arawaks, the disease took a wild and dangerous course in the uninitiated European hosts. Beginning as an ulcer, the "buba" was "painless, hard and blackish."[1] This was followed by "burning scabs, rashes, joint pains and gummy tumours the size of eggs or loaves of bread all over the body." In some cases it ate away the lips, nose, throat and tonsils, turning the face into "foul drippings."[2] Within a few weeks the victims were suffering intensely and within a year many were dead.

Supporting the theory of American origin are archeological findings in the United States, Mexico, Guatemala and Peru, where syphilis-like skeletal evidence was discovered in pre-Columbian bones.[2] It is known, though, that yaws and pinta, two other treponema illnesses long present in the New World, leave similar marks. The medicinal use of guaiac or guayacan, a tree native to the Indies, is cited as proof that syphilis originated in the place where nature provided the remedy.[1]

European Origin

Researchers who consider all venereal conditions as if one disease believe that syphilis existed in Europe before Columbus' travels. A European historian claims that syphilis had appeared sporadically in Europe long before 1494.[1] Some think that leprosy, which was so prevalent in European countries, was actually a variety of syphilis.[5]

In England a recent archeological excavation of a medieval friary has uncovered human remains preceding 1493 that are afflicted with the classic marks of syphilis. These bones have the typical "worm-eaten look" in the skull and destructive changes in the knees that characterize syphilis infection.[3]

Historians cite evidence of syphilis in ancient texts. "Scholars claimed to have identified the pox in the Babylonian poem of Gilgamesh, in the Eber papyrus, and in the ulceration of the genitals described by Paul of Aegina, Pliny the Younger, and so many others."[1] The Bible tells of Job, who had ulcerations and bone pains worse at night, symptoms of syphilis.

Other Treponemas: Yaws, Pinta, Bejel

Yaws, pinta, and bejel are varieties of treponema diseases that are not transmitted sexually and are not as contagious. These illnesses have been endemic for centuries and share the common symptoms of syphilis. Pinta, however, has distinct symmetrical blue patches on the face, hands and feet in the later stage. Unlike syphilis, these diseases tend to trade through casual skin contact, although it is thought that bejel can be transferred by sexual contact. The similarity of yaws, pinta and bejel to syphilis may explain the origin of syphilis-like symptoms in ancient skeletons uncovered in Europe and the Middle East. In past decades penicillin campaigns have been waged against venereal syphilis and yaws, resulting in their reduction or disappearance. The treponema illnesses are known to shift places. When venereal syphilis diminishes, yaws arises. In the areas where yaws has now disappeared, venereal syphilis has reappeared.[1] After moving to cool mountain areas from hot regions, people afflicted with yaws lose their sores and develop bejel.[4]

Symptoms – Then and Now

Early Appearances

In one of the oldest documents of the history of syphilis, a French military doctor describes early victims:

> The entire body is so repulsive to look at and the suffering is so great, especially at night, that this sickness is more horrifying than incurable leprosy or elephantiasis, and it can be fatal. He also saw sufferers who had lost their eyes, hands, noses, or feet during autopsy... he observed bones that were tumerous and suppurated to the marrow beneath... [1]

Many medical chronicles published in the 1500s delineate a routine order of symptoms. The primary pustules of "livid, black or whitish," surrounded by induration, show first, usually on the genitals. Then, a reddish rash, which looks similar to smallpox. A few days later all over the body appear "small protuberant nodules, from which a fetid sanies [discharge of serum, pus and blood] exudes." Sometimes greenish-black scabs congeal. Simultaneously, pains in the bones and joints are fierce.[1]

Next follows a quiescence of about a year, after which, "purulent tumours appear, along with bone like callosities, which are so painful at night that they make the sufferer scream." These growths form in the muscles or bones, "eating away cavities within them." Hard at first, they "soften into a whitish and viscous substance (gumma), they ulcerate the body extensively, exposing the bones and eating away at the nose, the lips, the palate, the larynx and the genitals." Remaining bones and limbs are "permanently twisted or stunted."[1]

Second Phase – Syphilis in the Sixteenth Century

After about 25 years the epidemic had vented some of its virulence, as one writer notes, "... the sickness has undoubtedly become weaker; the stench it causes is no longer so bad, and the ulcers are less obvious and less hard." Astutely, he recognizes, "... the venom still persists, insinuating its way into the body, where it gives rise to a variety of complaints."[1]

In 1546 a doctor observed, "... everyone is struck by the loss of the hair, and body hair in general,... some have no beards, others no eyebrows, others have bald heads."[1] The disease had begun an insidious transformation from a dramatic and powerful killer to an unseen and enduring adulterator of health.

In this attenuated state skin symptoms lessened in intensity while other symptoms became prominent. Hair loss was common, as was infection of the periosteum, leading to nightly occurrences of bone pain. The destructive properties remained, sacrificing eyes, hearing, palates and bones. Characteristic were the gummatous lesions that caused perforation and collapse of the nasal cartilage, indelibly marking the syphilis victim. Cachexia from severe suffering and sleeplessness occasionally led to death.[1]

Autopsies exposed lesions of the heart and aorta and of the brain and nervous system. After a 10 to 20 year hiatus, a third and deeper level of symptoms arose. Neurosyphilis resulted in various weaknesses and paralyses, such as locomotor ataxia (tabes) or paralysis of the accommodation muscles of the eye. Evidence of mental derangement from "meningoencephalitis of tertiary syphilis," is abundant: delusion of grandeur, dementia and suicidal madness.[1]

Congenital Symptoms

Paracelsus observed the congenital characteristics of syphilis, "... children, [who] catch the French sickness at the moment of conception, cannot free themselves from the infection, and... the disease grows with the child, revealing itself sooner or later by its power of corruption."[1] By one month of age the child shows early symptoms of "unpleasant nasal discharge, lesions on the skin and the mucous membranes and a general failure to thrive... "[3] In the 1800s syphilologists noticed distinct features in children which they named Hutchinson's triad: nerve deafness, interstitial keratitis and dental deformation. Also noted were infantile epilepsy, hydrocephaly, intellectual retardation, chorea and convulsions and the signal sign in babies, a sickly, emaciated infant with a head like an old man's.[1]

Freud wrote about the effects of hereditary syphilis in "Three Essays on the Theory of Sexuality":

> In more than half of the severe cases of hysteria, obsessional neurosis, etc., which I have treated, I have observed that the patient's father suffered from syphilis which had been recognized and treated before marriage, whether there was evidence of tabes or general paralysis, or whether the

> anamnesis indicated in some other way the presence of syphilitic disease. I should like to make it perfectly plain that the children who later became neurotic bore no physical signs of hereditary syphilis, so that it was their abnormal sexual constitution that was to be regarded as a last echo of their syphilitic heritage.[1]

Syphilis Symptoms in the Twentieth Century

In 1905 pathobiologists identified the Treponema pallidum, a member of the spiral-shaped, highly mobile and quick-dividing spirochete family, as the bacterial agent of syphilis. Scientists cannot study these fragile bacteria outside of the body, hence there is much mystery about their behavior. Diagnosis is made indirectly by detecting the presence of antibodies.

The organism replicates rapidly, within 30 hours, and spreads throughout the body via the lymphatic system. Able to cross the blood-brain barrier, it can enter into the brain, the cerebral spinal fluid and the eyeball. The spirochetes mostly stay in the extracellular fluid, but can breach cell membranes to live inside cells. When they are within the cells, treponema are undetected by serological testing and are unresponsive to penicillin.[7]

The first symptom usually noticed is on the skin: a round ulceration or chancre at the point of contact, which disappears in a few weeks. Indurated and swollen glands develop and persist for several months. Secondary symptoms appear in 2 months to 3 years: roseola, painless lesions of the mucous membranes, alopecia, uveitis, papilledema, aching pains in bones and joints, malaise, anorexia, nausea, meningitis, hepatitis, kidney and spleen disease.

From 5 to 30 years later tertiary symptoms occur in several categories: gummatous lesions with destruction of the palate, nasal septum, pharynx and larynx; deep boring pains in bones and joints. Cardiovascular lesions, aortitis, aortic aneurysm and valvular insufficiency. Meningovascular neurosyphilis with vertigo, malaise, seizures, aphasia, hemiplegia, weakness and wasting of shoulder and arm muscles, spastic paraplegia and sudden transverse myelitis. Parenchymatous neurosyphilis with tremors, convulsions, aphasia, hemiparesis, memory weakness, frequent weeping, temper tantrums, depression, mutism, delusions of grandeur, delusions they are dead, that their blood has ceased to circulate, that there is no blood, that their bodies are utterly destroyed. Tabes dorsalis (locomotor ataxia) with lightning pain in legs, wide gait, unsteadiness of gait, worse in the dark; sensation of walking on foam rubber, hyperesthesia, paresthesia; loss of bladder sensation, urine retention, incontinence, infections; impotence; hallucinatory paranoia, confusion, dementia, agitation; delusions of persecution, of having committed crimes.[8]

Treatment of Syphilis

Renaissance society viewed syphilis as a shameful, stigmatizing, terrifying disease, as is apparent by the treatment of its victims. Cities practiced a crude fashion of quarantine, rounding up all of the infected and banishing them to isolated islands or outside city walls. Hospitals denied access, relegating the afflicted to the streets, lunatic asylums and prisons. Doctors were horrified by the illness and most refused to treat its sufferers, leaving them in the hands of the less skilled "surgeons" and charlatans.

Besides caustics and hot iron cautery, mercury salve combined with steaming was the most common topical treatment. Daily the salve was rubbed vigorously into the ulcers and the patient placed in a high temperature steam bath. After 20 to 30 days, the feeble patient would develop swollen ulcers in his mouth and throat, purulent gums, loosened teeth and inevitably a profuse stream of foul-tasting saliva, symptoms of mercury poisoning. For centuries mercury had been used for skin diseases and leprosy, but it was unsuccessful in curing syphilis and caused numerous deaths from heart attacks, dehydration or poisoning. Nevertheless, "every adult European soon learned that five minutes with Venus" meant "a lifetime with Mercury."[2]

More frightened of the mercury treatment than the illness itself, victims sought other cures. Guaiac tea appeared early as an alternative, all the more popular because the decoction was prepared from the Guaiac tree, native to Hispanolia, the reputed source of the syphilis epidemic.

Both treatments endorsed the doctrine that treatment of syphilis was a way for man to atone for his sins against God, either through guaiac's "penitential fasting" or mercury's "expiatory purge."[1] Eventually, the roots, china smilax, sarsaparilla and sassafras replaced mercury and guaiac. Arsenic was given externally and internally, also gold, platinum, silver, antimony and bismuth. In the 19th century physicians understood that syphilis was a clinical illness. Charities founded hospitals specifically for syphilis patients and health officials advocated for personal and institutional hygiene.

In 1917 a Viennese doctor detected that naturally acquired malaria would cause the symptoms of cerebral syphilis to disappear. He infected his patients with malaria to rid them of the disease. Until the discovery of penicillin, this was thought to be the only cure for syphilis.[9]

1943 marked a major innovation in the treatment of syphilis when American doctors first treated patients with the newly developed penicillin. The United States launched a worldwide crusade to eliminate syphilis. Cases of syphilis in all stages, including congenital and hereditary, responded to this treatment, and declined to an all-time low level. Ten years later, the incidence of syphilis rose in all countries and returned to pre-penicillin levels.[1] Today, penicillin remains the preferred conventional medicine, administered on diagnosis, even though a mid-1900's study shows that 60 to 70 percent of untreated cases never progress to develop latent syphilis symptoms.[1]

Hahnemann: Theory and Treatment

Hahnemann's understanding of the energetic rather than local nature of illness brought him to a concept of the infectious process and treatment of syphilis that was very different from other physicians of his time. Commonly, doctors would excise the syphilitic chancre in an attempt to end the condition. Hahnemann realized that the disease was present in the organism prior to the appearance of the chancre. In fact, he knew that the chancre appeared as a vicarious symptom of the larger illness.

> For in the spot, into which at the impure coition the syphilitic miasma had been first rubbed in and had been caught, it is, in the same moment, no more local; the whole living body has already received (perceived) its presence, the miasma has already become the property of the whole organism.
>
> There is not to be perceived, indeed, any morbid transmutation in that spot during the first days, but the specific venereal transformation takes place in the internal of the body irresistibly, from the first moment of infection until syphilis has developed itself throughout the whole body, and only then (not before), nature, loaded down by the internal malady, brings forth the local symptom peculiar to this malady, the chancre, usually in the place first infected; and this symptom is intended by nature to soothe the internal completed malady.[10]

So effective is the skin symptom, that patients who had no external manipulation of this symptom were protected from further progression of syphilis. Hahnemann reported that in his 50 years of treating syphilis he had never seen a patient with an untreated chancre develop a full blown case of the venereal disease.[10]

The Syphilitic Miasm

Hahnemann concluded that mankind's illnesses are the consequence of miasms, psora, sycosis and syphilis, inherited derivatives of potent ancestral diseases. He believed that the syphilitic miasm developed because of aggressive treatments administered to the syphilis chancre. This suppression robs the organism of its outward expression of illness and directly weakens the individual.

Although no one elucidates the hereditary nature of syphilis as clearly as Hahnemann, other physicians and medical writers emphasize the miasmatic potential of syphilis. Sanchez in 1785 refers to the latent appearance of symptoms as "... chronic venereal disease. The symptoms may disappear following medication, but the poison can remain, and can even be transmitted from father to son. The insidious disease can thus pass from generation to generation, showing itself only by chronic diseases, eye pains, or crooked shoulders or backs..."[1]

A character in a 19th century novel, contracts syphilis and contemplates its horrors:

> And he had a sudden vision of humanity ceaselessly tormented by the age-old virus. Since the beginning of the world, from father to son, all creatures passed on the immutable legacy, the eternal disease which had ravaged man's ancestors, which had even burrowed into the now-exhumed bones of ancient fossils! It had come down inexhaustible, through the centuries; today it still raged, concealing itself behind the symptoms of migraines, bronchitis, vapours and gout; from time to time it would surface, preferring to attack those who were poorly looked after and poorly fed... [1]

Voltaire wrote a fable in which "two sisters governed the world: smallpox and syphilis." The sisters lived apart for five thousand years, the elder one "spoiling people's looks and making war on beauty" and the younger, "a resident of snake-infested lands in the Americas, made a direct attack on everything that makes beauty useful and precious." "They paid each other visits" in the 15th century and "for ever since that time they seem to have resolved to live together for evermore."[2]

Syphilis Today

Syphilis cases declined in the decade after World War II with the advent of penicillin treatment. Health officials spoke of the eradication of the disease, pointing out the

decrease in both primary and congenital cases. The lack of threat of syphilis infection may have encouraged the sexual liberation of the 1960s and 1970s, but syphilis revitalized as a result.[7] 1960 saw an increase in cases, which peaked towards the 1980's and has since plateaued.
A large contingent of patients with symptomless syphilis has contributed to altering the form of syphilis. "In the 1950s and 1960s the primary and secondary cases declined, but there was an increase in the number of latent ones which were a fertile source of later disease... "[7] Physicians in 1968 forewarned: "Numerous cases of secondary syphilis are now being seen with a few cutaneous manifestations or with an atypical appearance.
In the absence of characteristic skin lesions, early secondary syphilis may become manifest as a bizarre syndrome, or it may mimic many systemic diseases."[7]

The conclusion is that syphilis has never been eliminated but has only been disguised, as Fracastoro foretold five centuries ago: "And this disease of which I speak, this syphilis too, will pass away and die out, but later it will be born again and be seen again by our descendants just as in bygone ages we must believe it was observed by our ancestors."[7]

AIDS and Syphilis

The onset of AIDS in the early 1980s recalls the initial outbreak of syphilis. AIDS burst upon the scene with suddenness and fierceness in a population group known to have promiscuous sexual conduct. The early cases deteriorated rapidly to death. Now AIDS has mutated into a chronic illness similar to modern secondary syphilis, with an enormous medley of "imitator" symptoms and a dormancy in the appearance of other symptoms.[7]

Scientists speculate that suppression of active syphilis infection has led to immune system vulnerability, thus laying the groundwork for AIDS.[7] Because treponema affects the thymus gland, the immune system weakens, leading to vulnerability, illness and collapse.

Mitchell reports that syphilis has transformed due to the erroneous decision of doctors to use benzathine penicillin G as the conventional treatment. This antibiotic is an efficient medication because it is injected in one dose and remains in the serum for up to 12 weeks. However, penicillin G is bactericidal only in the initial stage of treponema's growth and is not able to pass the blood-brain barrier. By three weeks, when the infected patient notices the chancre and goes for treatment, the treponema has entered all areas of the body, including the central nervous system. Penicillin G, administered at this time, eradicates the bacteria in the blood and results in negative follow-up serum tests. Meanwhile, the spirochetes in the cerebral spinal fluid have not been touched.[11]

Noting that recurrent infections of syphilis in the male homosexual community were treated with repeated doses of penicillin G, Mitchell concludes, "While the bacterium was removed from their peripheral blood system and their symptoms were abated, their central nervous systems underwent countless untreated invasions of TP. The 1960s and 1970s provided two decades of neurological inbreeding of this infection. It is little wonder that today we find ourselves in an AIDS epidemic so similar to the malignant syphilis epidemic of the 1400s."[11]

Coulter posits that AIDS is a metamorphosis of syphilis, in which the treponema has exercised its natural ability to resist extermination. "Thus a major cause of the present AIDS epidemic has undoubtedly been the masking of syphilis by antibiotic abuse, suppressing the disease and causing it to smolder away for decades like an underground fire."[7] He cites physicians who noticed the curious decline of serologically diagnosed syphilis cases along with the dramatic increase of AIDS cases.[7] One of these doctors declares, "AIDS is simply a new face, a new disguise, a new chemical environment for syphilis – an old and infinitely resourceful enemy."

The possible relationship between syphilis and AIDS clarifies the perplexing geographical distribution of AIDS. Haiti and several African nations that exhibit a greater number of AIDS cases also report a high incidence of endemic syphilis. Moreover Haiti, which is on the island of Hispaniola, has had endemic yaws for centuries, predating Christopher Columbus' Caribbean contact 500 years ago.[7]

Political, Social and Literary Influence

Political Effects

"For five centuries now syphilis has meddled in the politics, wars, literature and sex lives of the civilized world... Civilization and syphilization have always been one and the same."[2]

Syphilis has had a heavy political impact. It played no favorites, so that kings and rulers such as King Francis I and King Henry VIII, were afflicted together with their subjects. King Henry's daughter, "Bloody Mary," contracted congenital syphilis and displayed its striking symptoms in her appearance: "face prematurely old and scarred; thin, moth-eaten hair; square head with grotesquely protruding forehead." She died prematurely at age 42 due to syphilitic aneurysm.[14] The decline of Valois France and of Ottoman Turkey has been traced to their royal rulers contracting syphilis.[15] Ivan the Terrible may have been acting out his syphilitic taint when he committed violent assaults on his enemies.

Jean Paul Marat, the murderous dictator of the French Revolution, embodied many syphilitic characteristics. An anarchist opposed to all systems of royal governing, he used his power ruthlessly, advocating rule by terror. Described as "5 feet tall, broad and bony head,... his eyes [were] not on the same horizontal line because one of his cheekbones was higher than the other... He inspired repugnance, disgust and contempt... Unprepossessing in appearance, violent in manner, egotistic in outlook... suspicion present to a pathological degree. Within him was the seed of violence which later was to become the Terror."[16]

Marat was known for his grandiose writing:

> I have unmasked the Parisian general, raised the army and the fleet against their despotic chiefs... I have struggled against oppressors of every kind; I have rescued a hundred thousand victims from judicial tyranny... I have been pursued again and again by the ministers and municipal administrators. Twenty military expeditions directed against me – this kind of life,... which freezes the most callous heart, I have led for 18 long months... without blanching at the sight of the sword always pointed at my heart.[16]

A knife to the heart killed Marat. It was wielded by a young woman who entered his apartment by deception. She found Marat in his bath soothing his pruritis (dermatitis herpetiformis) and stabbed him.

Throughout history syphilis has profited from the circumstances of wars and battles and may have influenced their outcomes. Some besieged countries used syphilis as a hidden defence, allowing their infected prostitutes to sleep with enemy soldiers and waiting for the subsequent symptoms to enfeeble the invaders. During his brutal conquer of Mexico in search of gold, it is reputed that Fernando Cortez and his soldiers intentionally infected the native women with syphilis. He knew that the disease would be passed to the men and the ill defenders would succumb easily to his invading forces. Other armies, such as Napoleon's, contracted syphilis unwittingly and weakened their own ranks and fighting ability.

In World War I nearly twenty percent of allied soldiers were infected with syphilis, rising to epidemic proportions and spreading to civilian populations.[7] After the war fear of contracting syphilis was at an hysterical pitch, calming down only after the production of penicillin during World War II. "In the general scheme of things, syphilis is no more than a sign or warning that human politics, economics or war have concentrated a lot of homeless and unhappy men or women in one place."[2]

Social Effects

Since its appearance in Europe, syphilis has been associated with prostitutes. Prostitution and liberal sexual standards, especially for men, were an accepted part of society for many centuries. Brothels and brothel districts were a way to protect virtuous women from men, who were satiating their natural desires. After the appearance of syphilis, sex became associated with death and disease and prostitutes became the symbols of shame.[9] Victims of the disease, especially women, were punished rather than cared for. In the 18th century, after forced medical treatment, prostitutes were beaten by doctors and nurses as punishment for catching the disease.[2]

The reaction of society was to conceal syphilitic symptoms with wigs, perfume and heavy makeup and to advocate abstinence or stringent sexual conduct. In this atmosphere Puritanism gained a stronghold. Some sociologists believe that Puritanism played a biological selection role in European societies by ensuring "stern morals" prohibiting "fornication and adultery" and producing the probability of "a long life... and a large and healthy progeny."[9] The dying out of noble families, whose morals were laxer than the lower classes, "fostered an upward social mobility which facilitated Europe's cultural innovation."[9]

"Witch hunts," which arose in the 16th and 17th centuries, are thought to have been in part a projection of society's guilt, anger and shame about syphilis.[9] Vulnerable women suffered persecution, while male victims of syphilis excused their sexual behavior as the result of bewitchment. The rise and decline of witch hunts parallels the epidemic pattern of malignant syphilis.

The advent of penicillin and its success as a treatment of syphilis turned the disease from a social and moral transgression into a public health campaign. Epidemiologists began to track victims and their sexual contacts. Advertisements urged prophylaxis and early treatment and syphilis lost its anxiety-filled image and social stigma.

Literary Effects

> But the one [disease] which is most a part of our culture, the one which has terrorized people the most, the one which has had the greatest influence on morality and literature, is unquestionably syphilis. It killed fewer people

> than tuberculosis, or even alcoholism, and it was less feared than any form of psychosis, and yet it was the disease which caused the most, and the blackest, ink to flow.[1]

Girolamo Fracastoro, a papal physician and poet, in 1530 published an acclaimed epic poem on the nature of syphilis. The poem, "Syphilis Sive Morbus Gallicus," recounted the plight of a poor shepherd boy, Syphilis (hog lover). The poem is remarkable as much for its medical accuracy as its literary quality. Fifteen years later Fracastoro wrote a treatise on the epidemiology of syphilis, noting its changing character and proposing that it was spread by "tiny invisible living things."[1]

Fracastoro had an unusual start in life. It is said that he was born with his "mouth... closed so that surgery was obliged to separate the lips." Later, "... his mother was killed by lightening while she held him safely in her arms."[18]

Early accounts describing the horrifying symptoms of syphilis were soon succeeded by literary treatises, poetry and plays, as writers began to contemplate and process the effects of syphilis upon the psyche of society. In 1524 Erasmus wrote a satire on syphilis in which Gabriel compares syphilis to the plague and decides that the plague is less cruel because it kills instantly. "But what is syphilis if not an unending death?"[1] Syphilis was an important background topic in Shakespeare's plays. His characters worried about contracting the disease, and made political puns about those who wore wigs to hide their hair loss.

The poems and novels of authors who had syphilis themselves often convey the influence of the disease. Retribution is the theme of a Maupassant novella. After war a soldier returns from war to find his love Irma in hospital with syphilis. She explains that the "Prussian bastards" raped her and "they have poisoned me." Asked why she did not seek treatment, a spark of fire comes into Irma's eyes: "No, I wanted to have my revenge, even if it killed me! And I have poisoned them too, all of them, all, as many as I could."[1]

Oscar Wilde wrote *The Picture of Dorian Gray* while he was developing the neurological symptoms of syphilis. In the novel, Dorian remains young and beautiful while his portrait, hidden upstairs in a locked room, deteriorates with every cruel and heartless act that he commits.[20]

"Many scholars are of the opinion that for some individuals syphilis can entail a brief but enormous increase in their intellectual and creative powers. As examples I need only name Nietzsche and Hugo Wolf or Maupassant, Heine and Baudelaire, Beethoven... "[21] Nietzsche, the 19th century philosopher, allegedly contracted syphilis as a young adult.

During his most productive and revolutionary period of philosophical thinking and writing, Nietzsche's became extremely isolated, eventually falling into mental collapse, suicidal depressions, incoherence and confusion. He wrote to a colleague, "In the end I would have much preferred being a Basle professor to being God... " One year before Nietzsche's death a friend found him in a public marketplace, embracing a horse.[22]

The influence of syphilis on literature and the arts is best summed up by Marc La Marche:

Syphilis

Are you not, Syphilis, the great go-between
Working to put man in touch with his genius,
The source of powerful thoughts, the transmitter
Of the seeds of art and science, the inspirer
Of delightful follies?

Crush with sobs the lyrical breast
Of the sublime musician
Inspire the weary metaphysician,
Shape the harrowed eye of the wretched painter
And the voice of the tragedian.
The world still awaits torches and kings,
The ambassadors of the Chimera.
You can give them to us... If we must put up crosses
To get them, we accept your laws
O Syphilis, salt of the Earth![1]

Appendix B

Bibliography

Works Cited 'Dynamic Materia Medica'

Dust Jacket: Schneider, M S. *A Beginner's Guide to Constructing the Universe.* New York: HarperCollins, 1994.

Pg v: Campbell, J. *The Hero With a Thousand Faces.* New York: Penguin Books, 1959.

Introduction

Pg. 2: Hobhouse, Rosa Waugh. *Life of Christian Samuel Hahnemann, Founder of Homoeopathy*. CW Daniel Company, 1933.

Perceiving Material Medica

Pg. 8: Hahnemann, Samuel. *Organon of Medicine. 6th ed.* trans. By W. Boericke. (New Delhi: B. Jain Publishers, 1992.

Pg. 11: Allen, T F. *The Encyclopedia of Pure Materia Medica.* ReferenceWorks, 2001.

Pg. 12: Emerson, R W. *Self-Reliance and other Essays*. Mineola, NY: Dover Publications, 1993.

Pg. 16: Schneider, M S. *A Beginner's Guide to Constructing the Universe.* New York: HarperCollins, 1994.

Pg. 18: Hahnemann. *Organon.*

Fracastoro

Pg. 23: Eatough, Geoffrey. *Fracastoro's 'Syphilis'.* Liverpool: Francis Cairns, 1984, 288-334, 338-44, 349-52, 354-65.

Pg. 25 Eatough, 212-16, 312-8, 173-6.

Androctonus Amoreuxi Hebreus

Pg. 28: Sherr, J. "Androctonus amoreuxii hebraeus"in *Dynamic Provings, Vol 1.* England: Dynamis Books, 1997.

Pg. 38: The Bible. Bible Scholar Computer Program, Israeli Research Society, 1992.

Aurum Metallicum

Pg. 42: Allen, T.F.
Van Zandvoort, R. *The Complete Repertory.* v.4.5 MacRepertory.
Pg. 44: *The Bible.*

Haliaeetus Leucocephalus

Pg .54: Sherr, J. "Haliaeetus leucocephalus" in *Dynamic Provings, Vol 1.*
Pg. 54: Tennyson, A. "The Eagle," in Kennedy, X J. An Introduction to Poetry, 7th ed. New York: HarperCollins Publishers, 1990.
Pg. 60: Black, Cynthia, ed. *The American Eagle.* Oregon: Beyond Words Publishing, 1994, 72.
Pg. 68: *The Bible.*

Guaiacum

Pg. 74: Hahnemann, S. *Materia Medica Pura.* Reference Works, 2001.
Phatak, S R. *Materia Medica of Homeopathic Medicines.* Reference Works, 2001.
Vermeulen, F. *Synoptic Materia Medica.* Reference Works, 2001.
Van Zandvoort.
Pg. 86: Eatough, 146-74, 174-8, 184-99, 228-40, 4-6, 24-7, 31-54, 57-9, 80-2, 85-9, 380-400, 402-13.

Hepar Sulphuris Calcareum

Pg. 92: Kent, J T. "Hepar Sulphur" in *Lectures on Homeopathic Materia Medica.* Reference Works, 2001.
Pg. 98: Gladwin, F E. *The People of the Materia Medica World. A Comparative Materia Medica.* New Delhi: National Homoeopathic Pharmacy, 1974.

Mercury

Pg. 102: Allen, T F.
Pg. 104: Allen, T F.
Boericke, W. *Homeopathic Materia Medica.* Reference Works, 2001.
Clarke, J H. *Dictionary of Practical Materia Medica.* Reference Works, 2001.
Choudhuri, N M. *A Study on Materia Medica and Repertory.* Reference Works, 2001.

Farrington, E A. *Clinical Materia Medica.* Reference Works, 2001.
Hahnemann. *Materia Medica Pura.*
Hering, C. *Guiding Symptoms.* Reference Works, 2001.
Kent.
Phatak.
Roberts, H A. *Sensations "As If".* Reference Works, 2001.
Vermeulen.
Van Zandvoort.
Encarta Encyclopedia. Macintosh Edition, 1994.
Grolier Encyclopedia. Macintosh Edition, 2001.
Pg. 114: Internet URL: http://www.levity.com/alchemy/ripmerc.html
Pg. 115 internet URL: http://www.cs.mu.oz.au/research/mercury/information/doc-latest/reference_manual_1.html
Pg. 116: Internet URL: http://www.mercurysafety.co.uk/mercdent.ht
Internet URL: http://www.geocities.com/toothk/bernie4.html
Internet URL: http://www.lef.org/magazine/mag2001/may2001_report_mercury_2.html
Internet URL: http://www.lef.org/magazine/mag2001/may2001_report_mercury_2.html
Internet URL: http://www.geocities.com/toothk/bernie2.html
Internet URL: http://www.msund.is/heild/Heilbrigdi/Sjukdomsvaldar/Amalgam/Default.htm
Pg. 118: Eatough, 402-17, 424-8, 434-48, 455-8, 269-80.
Pg. 119: Bradford, The Pioneers of Homoeopathy. Philadelphia: Boericke & Tafel 1897.

Phytolacca

Pg. 124: Kent, J T. "Phytolacca," in *Lectures on Homeopathic Materia Medica.* Reference Works, 2001.

Platina

Pg. 175: Hahnemann, S. *Chronic Diseases.* Reference Works, 2001.
Pg. 182: Meyer, V, Dr. "Platina," *Proceedings of the American Institute of Homeopathy,* 219.
Pg. 183: Julian, O A. "Pathogenesis of Platinum 1980," *The British Homoeopathic Jl,* 72:1 (Jan, 1983) 31-51.

Stillingia Sylvatica

Pg. 192: Clarke.
Pg. 198: Allen, T F.
Pg. 203: Eatough, 309-24, 349-50, 366-71, 376-83.
Pg. 204: Lorca, FG. *Blood Wedding* trans.Ted Hughes. London: Faber and Faber, 1997.

Syphilinum

Pg. 208: Allen, H C. *Materia Medica of the Nosodes.* Reference Works, 2001.

Thallium

Pg. 232: Quetel, C. *The History of Syphilis*. Baltimore, Maryland: The Johns Hopkins University Press, 1990.
Pg. 234: Packard, F R. "References to Syphilis in the Plays of Shakespeare," *Annals of Medical History*, 1:2, 194-200.

Iridium to Plumbum

Pg. 240: Eatough, 379-412, 413-15.
Pg. 241: Quetel, C.

Conclusion

Pg 245: J Sherr, Dynamis School Lectures, "Homoeopathic Laws"

Syphilis The Disease

Pg. 250: Eatough, 245-54, 297-306, 319-78, 378-9.
Pg. 251: Berkow, R. ed. *Merck Manual of Diagnosis and Therapy*. Rahway, New Jerswey: Merck & Co., Inc., 1987.

Works Cited Thallium

1. Borges, T. *Thallium*. Chemical Hazard Evaluation Group, Biomedical and Environmental Information Analysis Section, Health Sciences Research Division, Oak Ridge National Laboratory, Oak Ridge, Tennessee. December, 1994.

2. "Thallium Poisoning in Guyana" – A National Crisis. *Lancet*, 1 (1987): 604.

3. Heal, S. "A Green Bud." Unpublished manuscript.

4. Medical Consequences of Conflict. *BMJ*; 316 (1998): 1852.

5. "Racists Planned to Poison Mandela".
Internet URL: http://www. connectcorp.net/~trufax/general/alert.html

6. Van der Stoel, M. "U.N. Report on the Situation of Human Rights in Iraq".
Internet URL: http://www.unhcr.ch/refworld/.un/chr/chr96/country/1996_61.html

7. "Iraqi Regime Using Poison to Silence Opposition".
Internet URL: www. neda.net/iran-wpd/vol1015/i1015-06.html

8. The "Use of Terror Against Ethnic Minorities in Iraq".
Internet URL: http://awesomeseminars.com/iraq/iraq4.html

9. Rasmussen, OV. "Thallium Poisoning: An Aspect of Human Cruelty." *Lancet* 1 (1981):1164.

10. "1999 Country Reports on Human Rights Practices Released by the Bureau of Democracy, Human Rights, and Labor U.S. Department of State," February 25, 2000 IRAQ Internet URL:
http://www.state.gov/www/global/ human_rights/1999_hrp_report/iraq.html

11. House of Commons Internet URL: http://www.parliament.the-stationery office.co.uk/pa/cm199293/cmhansrd/1993-04-02/Debate-1.html

12. Dabrowska, K. "Iraqi Intelligence Activities in Europe." Internet URL:
http://www.iraqfoundation.org/forum/vsandarts/2000/fjun/22_dabrowska.html

13. "DOE Openness: Human Radiation Experiments: Roadmap to the Project. Oral

Histories:" Medical Physicist Kathering L. Lathrop and Physician Paul V. Harper. Thallium Research.
Internet URL: http://tis.eh.doe.gov/ohre/roadmap/histories/0472/0472d.html

14. Abney, E. "Thallium Toxicology. Unpublished manuscript."

15. Bank, WJ. *Arch Neuro* 5 (1972): 456-64.

16. Dolgner, R. *Int Arch Occup. Environ Health*. 48 (1981): 375-89.
17. Berkow, R., ed. *The Merck Manual of Diagnosis and Therapy*. Rahway, New Jersey: Merck Sharp and Dohme Research Laboratories, 1987, 2563.

18. Clarke, JH. *Dictionary of Practical Materia Medica*. India: B. Jain Publishers, 1993, 1405.

19. Cavanagh, JB. *Neuropathol. Appl. Neurobiol.* 17 (1991): 3-9.

20. "Prussian Blue." Internet URL:
http://www.nlm.nih.gov/medlineplus/ druginfo/ prussianblueoral 202737.html

21. "Prussian Blue." Internet URL:
http://www.radsci.ucla.edu/ telemed/zhuling/treatment.html

22. "Milk thistle." Internet URL:
http://www.health-rewards.com/ herb_milk_thistle.html

23. Thallium and a Pale Horse, *The Lancet* (letter) 1 (1987): 872.

24. Internet URL: http://www.radsci.ucla.edu/telemed/zhuling/index.html

25. McConnell, M. "Rescue on the Internet". Internet URL:
http://www.readersdigest.com/rdmagazine/specfeat/archives/rescueint.html

26. McMillan, TM. *J Neurol Neurosurg Psychiatry* 63 (1997): 247-250.

Works Cited Syphilis the Disease

1. Quetel, C. *The History of Syphilis*. Baltimore, Maryland: The Johns Hopkins University Press, 1990.

2. Nikiforuk, *A. The Fourth Horseman*. New York: M. Evans & Company, Inc., 1991.

3. Miller, H. *Secrets of the Dead.* London: Macmillan Publishers Ltd, 2000.

4. Karlen, *A. Man and Microbes. Disease and Plagues in History and Modern Times.* New York: G.P. Putnam's Sons, 1995.
5. Packard, FR. "References to Syphilis in the Plays of Shakespeare," Annals of Medical History, 1:2, 194-200.

6. Arrizabalaga, J, Henderson, J and French, R. *The Great Pox. The French Disease in Renaissance Europe.* New Haven: Yale University Press, 1997.

7. Coulter, HL. *AIDS and Syphilis. The Hidden Link.* Berkeley, Ca: North Atlantic Books, 1987.

8. Berkow, R, ed. *Merck Manual of Diagnosis and Therapy. Rahway*, New Jersey: Merck & Co., Inc., 1987.

9. Andreski, S. *Syphilis, Puritanism and Witch Hunts.* New York: St. Martin's Press, 1989.

10. Hahnemann, S. *The Chronic Diseases*. India: B. Jain Publishers, 1993.

11. Mitchell, RB. *Syphilis As AIDS.* Austin, Texas: Edward-William Publishing Co., 1988.

12. Jones, JH. *Bad Blood. The Tuskeegee Syphilis Experiment.* NY: Free Press, 1981.

13. "The Lost Children of Rockdale County." Frontline, www.pbs.org.

14. Parran, T. *Shadow on the Land:* Syphilis. NY: Reynal and Hitchcock, 1937.

15. McNeill, W H. *People and Plagues.* Garden City, New York: Anchorage Books, 1976.

16. Scarlett, EP. "Jean Paul Marat. The Physician As Revolutionist." *Annals of Medical History.* 2:1 71-78.

17. Neville, K. *The Eight.* NY: Random House, 1990.

18. Van Wyck, W. *The Sinister Shepherd: A Translation of Girolamo Fracastoro's "Syphilidis Sive de Morbo Gallico Libri Tres."* Los Angeles: Primavera Press, 1934.

19. Pelensky, O. *Isak Dinesen: The Life and Imagination of a Seducer.* Athens: Ohio University Press, 1991.

20. Ellman, R. *Oscar Wilde.* NY: Vintage Books, 1987.

21. "The Vision of Sickness in Jens Bjorneboe's Writings."
Internet URL http://home.att.net/~emurer/about/Kierulf.htm

22. Beckman, T. "The Life of Nietzsche."
Internet URL http://www.ask.com/main/metaAnswer

Notes